OXFORD HANDBOOKS IN EMERGENCY MEDICINE
Series Editors   R. N. Illingworth, C. E. Robertson, and A. D. Redmond

OXFORD HANDBOOKS IN EMERGENCY MEDICINE

This series will cover topics of interest to all Accident and Emergency staff. The books are aimed at all junior doctors and at nurses, particularly those who deal with patients in the acute setting. Each book starts with an introduction to the topic, including epidemiology where appropriate. The clinical presentation and the immediate practical management of common conditions is described in detail, so that the casualty officer or nurse is able to deal with the problem on the spot. A specific course of action is recommended for each situation, and alternatives discussed.

The Management of Head Injuries

David G. Currie
Consultant Neurosurgeon
Aberdeen Royal Infirmary

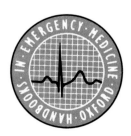

Oxford • New York • Tokyo
OXFORD UNIVERSITY PRESS
1993

Oxford University Press, Walton Street, Oxford OX2 6DP
Oxford   New York   Toronto
Delhi   Bombay   Calcutta   Madras   Karachi
Kuala Lumpur   Singapore   Hong Kong   Tokyo
Nairobi   Dar es Salaam   Cape Town
Melbourne   Auckland   Madrid
and associated companies in
Berlin   Ibadan

Oxford is a trade mark of Oxford University Press

Published in the United States
by Oxford University Press Inc., New York

A catalogue record for this book is available from the British Library

Library of Congress Cataloging in Publication Data
The Management of head injuries / David G. Currie.
(Oxford handbooks in emergency medicine ; 5)
Includes bibliographical references and index.
1. Head—Wounds and injuries.   I. Series.
[DNLM: 1. Head Injuries—therapy—handbooks. 2. Brain Injuries—
therapy—handbooks. WB 39 098 v.5 1993]
RD521.M347   1993   617.5'1044—dc20   93–3454

ISBN 0–19–262385–0 (hbk)
ISBN 0–19–262052–5 (pbk)

Typeset by Footnote Graphics, Warminster, Wiltshire
Printed in Great Britain on acid-free paper by
Biddles Ltd., Guildford & Kings Lynn

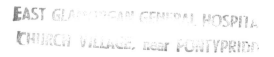

Preface

Head injury is a common problem, and one which is dealt with very largely by non-specialists, often by junior doctors and often in district hospitals where specialist neurosurgical assistance is lacking. This book is intended to be a guide for the junior doctor working in the Accident and Emergency Department or the Orthopaedic or General Surgical Ward. The emphasis is on the early management of the head-injured patient. The section on 'Operative surgery' has been written in the knowledge that the isolated General Surgeon may, on occasions, be required to operate on head-injured patients when transfer to a specialist centre is impossible.

This is very much a practical handbook, and not a substitute for the excellent textbooks on the subject which are currently available and are referred to in the notes on Further reading.

Aberdeen   D.G.C.
February 1993

Drug dosages have been included for many drugs. While great care has been taken to ensure the accuracy of the book's content when it went to press, neither the authors nor the publisher can be responsible for the accuracy and completeness of the information. If there is any doubt, the British National Formulary, manufacturers' current product literature, or other suitable reference should be consulted.

Contents

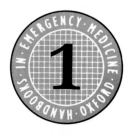

Chapter 1

Introduction

Epidemiology

In Scotland, with a population of approximately 5 million people, 80 000 to 90 000 patients are seen each year following injuries to the head. This gives an attendance rate of 1600 to 1800 per 100 000 of the population. The attendance rate in the United States is almost double this figure. Head-injured patients are seen initially by junior doctors in Accident and Emergency Departments in district general hospitals and teaching hospitals, and by General Practitioners in community hospitals. On the basis of this initial assessment approximately 20 000 patients are admitted to hospital annually in Scotland. A similar proportion, 300 to 400 per 100 000 of the population, is admitted to hospital in England and Wales. The patterns of aetiology, attendance rate, and admission rate vary in other European countries, as does the influence of alcohol. There is a wide variation in the nature of the admitting unit, which may be in a small isolated district hospital on the one hand or in a major teaching hospital on the other.

The care of head-injured patients is by General Surgeons, Orthopaedic Surgeons, and Accident and Emergency specialists in most instances. Only a minority are admitted directly to Neurosurgical wards. In Scotland, less than 1000 patients are eventually admitted to Neurosurgical Units annually, and only a minority of this group require operative intervention by a Neurosurgeon. This means that only 1 per cent of all head-injured patients seen in the Accident and Emergency Department are admitted to Neurosurgical Units.

It is clear from these figures that a great deal of the decision-making in the management of head injuries is done by non-specialists, and often by junior doctors in a variety of specialties. Given the ratio of Neurosurgeons and Neurosurgical beds to population in the United Kingdom, head-injured patients will continue to be cared for in this fashion, and the quality of service provided depends crucially on the education of non-specialists in the early assessment and subsequent management of the head-injured patient. The main possibilities for improvement in our management of head injuries lie not in the area of operative neurosurgery but in the organization of the early management of the patient in the Accident and Emergency Department, in the admitting ward, and in transit between the admitting unit and the specialist centre.

The doctor with primary responsibility for head injuries is faced with a series of decisions.

Box 1.1 Decisions facing the doctor with primary responsibility for head injuries

- Who should have a skull X-ray?
- Who should be admitted to hospital?
- Who is at risk of an intracranial haematoma?
- Who should have a CT scan?
- Who should be transferred to a specialist centre?
- Who should be operated on at the base hospital?
- Who should be ventilated?

The doctor on the spot is also faced with certain practical tasks, and may not always have the benefit of specialist advice immediately to hand. The assessment and resuscitation of the head-injured patient are the task of the receiving doctor in the Accident and Emergency Department, and cannot be deferred until specialist help is available. The interpretation of skull X-rays and the management of scalp injuries also fall to the doctor on the spot, and in some circumstances the skull injury and even the intracranial haematoma may need to be dealt with by the non-specialist.

Causes of head injury

- **Road-traffic accidents**   **Sports injuries**   **Alcohol and head injury**

Head injuries are twice as common in men as in women. The great majority of head injuries are caused by road-traffic accidents, falls, and assaults; but the proportion of injuries due to each cause varies according to age-group. Falls and domestic accidents are much more common in the elderly, whereas assaults and industrial injuries are more common amongst younger men. Alcohol is the single commonest causative factor in head injury.

The aetiology of the accident is important in drawing attention to the possibility of associated injuries, and may be of medico-legal significance in an era of increasing litigation. It is essential to ask how the patient came to fall and strike the head. Where no obvious explanation is forthcoming it is possible that the accident was preceded by loss of consciousness, and this will require investigation in its own right. The fall may have been the result of a fit, a cardiac arrhythmia, or an intracranial haemorrhage. The account of an eyewitness is important in establishing how the accident happened; and when an immediate eyewitness is not available the observations of the police or other emergency personnel may be helpful. Occasionally, for instance, a driver may be involved in a road-traffic accident because of prior loss of consciousness. The police observations at the scene of the accident may raise this possibility. As well as supplying an explanation for the injury, the police, the ambulance crew, or other witnesses may be able to give valuable information about the patient's state of consciousness after the injury.

Box 1.2 Causes of head injury

- Road-traffic accidents
- Falls
- Domestic accidents
- Recreational accidents
- Industrial accidents
- Assault
- Fits and other causes of loss of consciousness

The nature of the head injury may also draw attention to the possible complications. The drunken patient, for instance, who falls forward and presents with a bleeding nose and black eyes is a prime candidate for an anterior cranial fossa fracture and CSF rhinorrhoea. The same injury may be complicated by a hyperextension injury of the neck and spinal-cord trauma. A recent study of head-injured patients with altered consciousness at the time of admission to a Neurosurgical Unit has compared those injuries caused by high-velocity impacts (as in road-traffic accidents) with those caused by low-velocity impacts (as in falls). In the case of high-velocity injuries there was a high incidence of multiple injuries, and, hence, a high incidence of extracranial complications, but only a 26 per cent incidence of intracranial haematoma. In the case of low-velocity injury the incidence of extracranial complications was much lower, but the incidence of intracranial haematoma was 59 per cent.

Head injury accounts for 26 per cent of all deaths due to injury in the United States and 2 per cent of all deaths. Head injuries account for only 1 per cent of all deaths in the United Kingdom. Some 57 per cent of all deaths from head injury in the United States are due to road-traffic accidents, and 12 per cent to falls. There is a bimodal distribution of deaths from head injury according to age-group, with the peaks occurring in the age-range 15–24 on the one hand and in the age-range over 75 years on the other.

Road-traffic accidents

Road-traffic accidents remain the commonest cause of severe head injury, and often form a component of multiple injuries in the same patient. The associated injuries commonly result in respiratory impairment or hypovolaemia, which, in turn, exacerbate the brain injury. Furthermore, the effects of respiratory impairment and hypovolaemia may be prolonged if the patient is trapped in the vehicle. In these circumstances it may be that a substantial proportion of the brain injury is due to systemic factors causing cerebral ischaemia and hypoxia, and only a relatively small part to the head injury itself.

Legislation to make the use of seat-belts compulsory was introduced in Australia in 1970, with a dramatic reduction in both the death-rate from road-traffic accidents and the incidence of head injury. Seat-belt legislation was introduced in the United Kingdom in 1983. One year later the death-rate from road-traffic accidents had fallen by 25 per cent, and this was largely due to the prevention of severe head injuries. One study in Nottingham compared the incidence of injuries in the three months before the legislation with that in the subsequent three months. There was a fall in the incidence of head injury of more than 50 per cent, and a similar fall in the incidence of facial injuries. Compulsory seat-belt legislation has been repealed in certain states in the United States, and in each case there has been a marked increase in the incidence of head injury.

Not only has the death-rate fallen after seat-belt legislation, but there has been a change in the pattern of head injury resulting from road-traffic accidents. Before the widespread wearing of seat-belts the unrestrained driver or passenger was thrown forwards, striking the windscreen with the head. This resulted in complex injuries of the head and face, together with scalp and facial lacerations. Compound, comminuted, and often depressed frontal fractures were seen, and the brunt of the brain injury was received by the frontal lobes. Some of the energy of the impact was absorbed as the frontal bones were fractured, thereby diminishing the force applied to the brain. Such a patient might require exploration and elevation of the frontal fractures, debridement of the damaged brain, maxillo-facial surgery, and possibly a tracheostomy. The survivors were left with disfiguring facial scars and intellectual impairment. Some suffered visual loss due to optic-nerve injuries. The seat-belted vehicle occupant involved in a similar accident is spared the complex, disfiguring frontal and facial injuries; but the brain injury may, paradoxically, be more severe. As the head is brought abruptly to rest, the energy derived from the loss of momentum is transmitted to the brain, causing diffuse damage rather than the localized damage described above.

Motor cycles and pedal cycles

Approximately 5000 serious injuries amongst pedal cyclists occur each year in the United Kingdom, with a 75 per cent incidence of head injury. As a result there are approximately 300 deaths each year. Pedal cyclists are more likely to suffer head injuries than those involved in motor-cycle accidents, and those suffering from head injuries have a higher incidence of severe head injuries than motor cyclists. Experience in the United States, Germany, and Australia has shown that the use of cycling helmets brings about a very substantial reduction in serious head injury. The potential reduction in head injuries as a result of the use of cycling helmets has been estimated in different studies as being between 80 per cent and 90 per cent. Cycling accidents occur most frequently on main roads, and particularly at road junctions. Provision of cycle lanes or cycle tracks reduces the incidence of head injury.

Sports injuries

Head injury occurs in most sports. There is some discernible pattern from sport to sport. In contact sports such as football and rugby blunt head injury is caused by clashes of heads or kicks. Scalp and skull injuries are uncommon. Head injury is the commonest cause of death in climbing accidents; and since the head injury is so often fatal the numbers of head-injured climbers seen in hospital are surprisingly small, even in popular climbing areas. As in the case of road-traffic accidents, injuries in climbing accidents are often multiple. Horse-riding is the single most dangerous sport in the context of head injury. Some 33 per cent of equestrian accidents include head injuries, and in 1983 there were 12 deaths in the United Kingdom. Studies of equestrian head injuries have shown a significant reduction in serious head injuries when protective headgear is worn. A British Standard for riding hats has been established.

Sports injuries account for 20–30 per cent of children's head injuries. Surprisingly, the sport most frequently implicated in the United Kingdom is golf! The majority of children thus injured are struck as their friends swing the club. Skull fractures occur in the majority of these children, and in most cases these are depressed fractures requiring elevation.

Alcohol and head injury

Alcohol is an important factor both in the aetiology of head injury and as a complicating factor. It is particularly implicated in head injuries caused by falls and assaults, and in pedestrians injured in road-traffic accidents; but irrespective of the cause of injury alcohol intoxication is associated with a higher incidence of head injury than that found in sober victims of injury. In Finland 64 per cent of intoxicated patients presenting in Accident Departments have head injuries, compared with 17 per cent of sober accident victims. In Scotland 40–50 per cent of patients admitted to hospital after head injury have recently taken alcohol.

The intoxicated patient is more likely to vomit and aspirate gastric contents. It is difficult to assess the extent to which the patient's conscious level is due to the head injury and how much to ascribe to alcohol. It is not uncommon for the relatives of head-injured patients to attribute the victim's drowsiness or failure to wake the next morning to his or her overindulgence on the previous night—indeed, it is not unknown in Scotland for the patient to be left 'to sleep it off' for more than 24 hours before it is realized that there is more to the stupor than can be ascribed to a hangover.

Since alcohol consumption is so common amongst head-injury victims impaired consciousness should never be attributed to the effects of alcohol alone. There is a poor correlation between conscious state and blood or breath alcohol levels, but experience in Glasgow has been that consciousness is not impaired until blood-alcohol levels exceed 2g/litre.

Pathophysiology of head injury

- **Primary and secondary brain injury** **Pathology of primary brain injury** **Intracranial pressure and cerebral perfusion** **Cerebrovascular autoregulation**

It is necessary to be aware of some theoretical concepts in order to appreciate the requirements of the head-injured patient.

Primary and secondary brain injury

The **primary brain injury** is that which is inflicted at the time of impact. It ranges from the minor concussional injury with brief loss of consciousness to the severe brain injury with prolonged coma or severe focal damage. The damage is established at the time of the impact, and is not amenable to surgical treatment. Recovery takes place, partially or completely depending on the severity of the brain injury, provided that a suitable environment is created to enable healing to proceed unhindered.

The **secondary brain injury** may follow at any time after the impact, and is due to a variety of potentially preventable or reversible causes such as intracranial haemorrhage, impaired respiration leading to hypoxia and hypercapnia, and decreased cerebral perfusion due to hypotension. The essence of head-injury management is the prevention and treatment of these secondary insults to the injured brain; and it is, therefore, essential for the doctor caring for the head-injured to be able to recognize deterioration when it occurs. In some instances, the primary injury may be relatively trivial, but the delayed development of an intracranial haematoma may put the patient's life at risk.

Pathology of primary brain injury

The primary brain injury is either **closed** or **penetrating**. In the United Kingdom the majority of head injuries are due to blunt trauma, and penetrating head injuries are relatively rare. The latter are seen more frequently in warfare and where there is a high incidence of civil violence.

The energy of the blunt head injury dissipates through the brain causing diffuse damage, the severity and duration of which depends on the force of the blow.

The relatively minor injury resulting in a brief period of unconsciousness causes a physiological disturbance without extensive anatomical disruption. With increasing severity of injury there is anatomical disruption, with damage to axons and synapses, and small areas of haemorrhage resulting in prolonged periods of unconsciousness or death. This diffuse injury of the brain can occur without a direct impact if severe inertial forces are applied, as, for example, when the head abruptly comes to rest in the impact of a road-traffic accident. The same mechanism is responsible for the damage caused when children are forcibly shaken in the course of non-accidental injury.

The kinetic energy of the moving head is abruptly transformed as the head comes to rest, and a shock wave passes through the skull and brain. A certain amount of energy may be dissipated when the skull is fractured, thus reducing the energy transmitted to the brain. Since the kinetic energy of different tissues depends on the density of the tissue the energy-transfer to different structures leads to shearing forces and disruption of axons.

Blunt trauma is also capable of causing focal damage. At the site of the blow the transient deformity of the skull causes local contusion of the underlying brain, with patchy areas of haemorrhage and necrosis. This **cerebral contusion** is commonly also seen at the opposite side of the head from the site of the blow—the so-called **contre-coup injury** (Fig. 1.1). The patient who falls backwards, for instance, striking the occiput is commonly found to have contusions of the frontal lobes. As a result of the impact, the temporal lobes

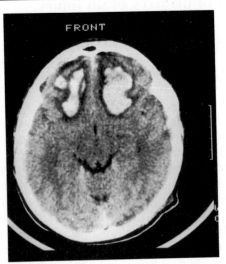

Fig. 1.1 • CT scan of bifrontal cerebral contusion caused by occipital head injury—'contre-coup' injury.

may be contused or frankly lacerated by the sharp edge of the sphenoid ridge anteriorly. Cerebral contusions are not static lesions, and following the injury there may be coalescence of areas of haemorrhage, and progressive swelling at the contused site may occur, giving rise to neurological deterioration.

The effect of the primary injury is recognized by the patient's state of consciousness and focal neurological deficit immediately after the impact. Thus the patient who is unconscious and has a hemiparesis at the scene of the accident is likely to have a diffuse concussional injury and a unilateral cerebral contusion. By contrast, the patient who is not knocked out, or is only briefly so, has had no significant primary injury, and any subsequent alteration in consciousness is due to some form of potentially reversible secondary insult.

Penetrating head injuries are often of low velocity, and do not usually impart the same high energy to the brain. Much of the force is expended in penetrating the skull, and the brain injury is localized. This is true also of low-velocity gunshot injuries such as are caused by handguns and air-rifles. High-velocity bullet injuries, on the other hand, cause severe diffuse damage.

Intracranial pressure and cerebral perfusion

The brain occupies an inelastic container, and any increase in the volume of the contents of the skull results in a rise in pressure. Cerebral perfusion depends on two factors—cerebral perfusion pressure (CPP) and cerebrovascular resistance. Cerebral perfusion pressure depends on systemic arterial blood-pressure (Fig. 1.2), while cerebrovascular resistance is determined by intracranial pressure (ICP). Cerebrovascular resistance may be increased by extracranial venous obstruction, as when the jugular veins are compressed in the neck or when venous return is impeded by tilting the patient head-down. A rise in intracranial pressure not accompanied by a rise in blood-pressure leads to reduced cerebral perfusion, as expressed in the equation CPP = BP − ICP. Cerebral perfusion pressure less than 40mm Hg results in a critical reduction in cerebral blood-flow.

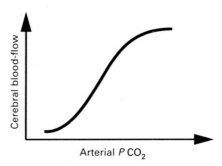

Fig. 1.2 • Effect of changes in $PaCO_2$ on cerebral blood-flow (CBF).

Rising pressure above the tentorium results in displacement of the brain in a caudal direction as the severity of the condition increases. The medial aspects of the temporal lobes eventually herniate through the tentorial hiatus. The upper brain stem is directly compressed, the medulla impacts in the foramen magnum, and the respiratory centre is rendered ischaemic. The herniating temporal lobe stretches the ipsilateral oculomotor nerve. Compression of the oculomotor nerve results in dilatation of the pupil, which finally fails to respond to light (Fig. 1.3).

In response to rising intracranial pressure, there is a reflex increase in systemic blood-pressure and slowing of pulse-rate—the Cushing reflex.

Increased intracranial pressure following head injury is caused by **diffuse swelling** or by **intracranial haematoma**, and sometimes by **CSF obstruction**, or by a combination of all these factors. Swelling of the brain is due to oedema or to increase in the cerebral blood volume. $PaCO_2$ has a very important influence on intracranial pressure. The cerebral arterioles are sensitive to changes in $PaCO_2$, dilating in response to a rise in $PaCO_2$ and constricting in response to a reduction in $PaCO_2$. The resulting change in intracranial blood volume leads to changes in intracranial pressure (Fig. 1.4). An increase in $PaCO_2$ from 5.3 kPa (40 mm Hg) to 10.6 kPa (80 mm Hg) leads to a doubling of the cerebral blood-

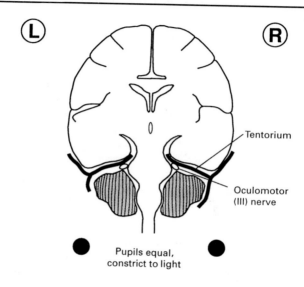

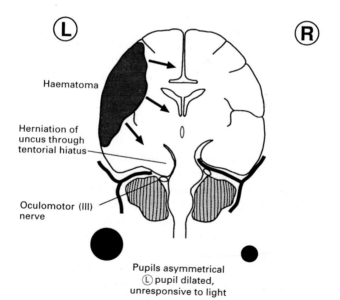

Fig. 1.3 • Mechanism of tentorial herniation due to intracranial haematoma.

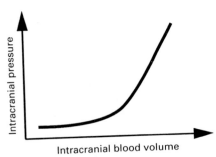

Fig. 1.4 • Relation of intracranial pressure (ICP) to intracranial blood volume.

flow and a reduction from 5.3 kPa to 2.6 kPa to a halving of the cerebral blood-flow. A rising $PaCO_2$ due to impaired ventilation in the head-injured patient leads to a rising intracranial pressure and impaired cerebral perfusion. Conversely, lowering the $PaCO_2$ by hyperventilation brings about a reduction in intracranial pressure, and is used to this end in the intensive management of severe head injuries. The critical importance of respiratory complications in the management of the head-injured patient will be referred to in subsequent chapters.

Cerebrovascular autoregulation

The arterioles of the cerebral circulation regulate cerebral blood-flow. In the healthy individual, the cerebral arterioles respond to systemic hypotension to as low as 60 mm Hg by dilating and maintaining a constant cerebral blood-flow. Conversely, systemic hypertension up to 160 mm Hg does not result in an increase in cerebral blood-flow because the cerebral arterioles constrict accordingly. This autoregulatory mechanism is impaired after injury to the brain, and a reduction in arterial blood-pressure may result in decreased cerebral blood-flow. The cerebral perfusion is vulnerable to fluctuations in systemic blood-pressure. The treatment of shock and blood loss is, therefore, a priority in the management of the severe head injury.

The measurement of conscious level

- **Glasgow Coma Scale** Verbal response Motor response Eye-opening response

It is of crucial importance to those caring for head-injured patients to be able to recognize changes in conscious level. This must be done in a precise and universally accepted fashion. Terms such as 'semi-conscious' or 'comatose' are not acceptable. The internationally accepted scale of consciousness is the **Glasgow Coma Scale** (Box 1.3).

Box 1.3	**Glasgow Coma Scale**	
		Score
Eyes	Spontaneously	4
Open	To speech	3
	To pain	2
	Do not open	1
Best	Orientated	5
verbal	Confused	4
response	Inappropriate words	3
	Incomprehensible sounds	2
	None	1
Best	Obeys commands	5
motor	Localizes to pain	4
response	Flexes limbs to pain	3
	Extends limbs to pain	2
	None	1
	Total	14

The scale is divided into three sections—the best verbal response, the best motor response, and the best eye-opening response.

Verbal response

The **verbal response** is recorded as orientated (in place, time, and person), confused (speaking in formed sentences but not orientated), inappropriate words (often expletives!), and incomprehensible sounds. Spurious results may be obtained if the patient is dysphasic.

Motor response

The **motor response** is recorded as obeying commands, localizing to painful stimuli, flexing the limbs in response to pain, extending the limbs, or no response. Suitable commands include 'put out your tongue' or 'hold up two fingers'. Placing the examiner's fingers in the palm of the patient's hand may elicit a grasp reflex, and give a false impression that the patient is obeying the command 'squeeze my fingers'. Some charts include a category—'withdrawal' or 'abnormal flexion'—in the motor response to pain. This addition to the original Glasgow Coma Scale is often difficult to define and poorly understood by those responsible for carrying out the recordings, and should be omitted. Purposeful movements such as pulling at the bedclothes, scratching, or attempting to remove the nasogastric tube are equivalent to localizing to a painful stimulus.

Eye-opening response

Record whether the patient opens the eyes spontaneously, in response to speech, in response to pain, or not at all.

An appropriate painful stimulus is achieved by applying pressure to the supraorbital nerve or applying pressure to the ear lobe. Pressing the nail-bed is not a suitable stimulus, since this will even elicit a response in the brain-dead patient, and the response, even in patients who are capable of localizing to a painful stimulus, is invariably to flex the limb.

A numerical value can be attached to each component of the scale, and the sum of the three recordings gives a Coma Score, which can be used to subdivide head-injured patients into groups according to conscious level. The maximum score in the fully conscious patient is 14.

The Coma Scale is one of the most important developments in the management of head injury. The Coma Scale makes it possible to recognize changes in consciousness reflecting recovery or deterioration. It is, therefore, a dynamic scoring system that must be reused at regular intervals. It enables the doctor with responsibility for the head-injured patient to give a precise description of the patient's conscious level to the neurosurgeon, and it provides one means of quantifying the severity of the injury. A modification of the scale is required in young children, and this is described in Chapter 8.

Further reading

Field, J. H. (1976). *Epidemiology of head injuries in England and Wales.* HMSO, London.

Jennett, Bryan and Teasdale, Graham (1981). *Management of head injuries,* Contemporary Neurology Series. F. A. Davis Co., Philadelphia.

Jennett, B., *et al.* (1978). Head injuries in three Scottish neurosurgical units. *British Medical Journal,* **2**, 955–8.

Jennett, B., *et al.* (1977). Severe head injuries in three countries. *Journal of Neurology, Neurosurgery, and Psychiatry,* **40**, 291–8.

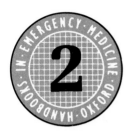

Chapter 2

Initial assessment

Key points in initial assessment

1 Most patients admitted to hospital after head injury are conscious and have no neurological deficit. They are admitted principally for observation, because the nature of their primary injury exposes them to delayed complications which may require prompt recognition and treatment.

2 In the unconscious patient it is vital to establish whether there has been a change in conscious level since the injury, as this may indicate a developing intracranial haematoma.

3 Severe headache and vomiting are indications for admission, as they may herald an intracranial haematoma or meningitis.

4 Any history of the consumption of alcohol or other drugs should be recorded, as should any bleeding or fluid discharge from nose or ears.

5 Absence of suitable supervision at home is an indication for observation in hospital.

6 The patient's state of alertness and conscious level should be recorded using the Glasgow Coma Scale.

7 By no means all head-injured patients require skull X-rays, and the main purpose of the skull X-ray is to determine whether the patient requires admission.

8 All patients with altered consciousness should have their blood sugar measured by the stick method.

9 The patient with a skull fracture who is not fully conscious has a 25 per cent chance of having a haematoma of some sort. In children 40 per cent of extradural haematomas occur without radiological evidence of a fracture.

10 The patient with CSF rhinorrhoea or otorrhoea should be admitted until the discharge has ceased or the fistula has been repaired.

11 The patient who has had a fit following injury may have further post-traumatic fits, and should be admitted for observation.

12 In head-injured patients with an impaired conscious level who are known to be affected by alcohol one must always assume that the impairment is due to the injury, and investigate or observe the patient appropriately.

In the case of the severely injured patient, and particularly the multiply injured patient, the first priority is to carry out a rapid assessment of the airway, breathing, and circulation, and to initiate resuscitation. However, of the very large number of patients seen every year in Accident and Emergency Departments following head injuries the great majority do not require admission, and a majority of those who do require admission are conscious and have no neurological deficit. These patients require to be admitted not because they have suffered a severe primary injury but because the nature of the injury exposes them to potentially serious complications. In order to recognize and treat delayed complications of the head injury promptly, these patients are admitted principally for observation. Only a minority have severe primary injuries, and the need for admission in this group is usually self-evident. The assessment and resuscitation of the patient with severe head injury is dealt with in Chapter 3.

The initial assessment, including the history, examination and investigations, should establish the following facts (Box 2.1).

Box 2.1 Facts to be established on initial assessment

- Has the patient had a head injury?
- Has the patient a scalp or skull injury requiring treatment?
- Does the patient require admission to hospital?

The history

The history should establish whether the patient has had a head injury. In some instances it may be clear that the patient collapsed because of some preceding loss of consciousness. It is important to establish how the injury happened. The circumstances of the injury indicate the severity of the blow, and draw attention to possible associated injuries. Where no clear history is available from the patient every effort should be made to interview relatives, ambulance crews, police, and other observers. In the case of the unconscious patient, it is particularly vital to establish whether there has been a change in conscious level since the time of the injury, indicating the possibility of a developing intracranial haematoma. If the patient was capable of talking at some stage after the injury the primary brain injury cannot have been severe. The time of the accident should be established. The greater the interval between injury and admission the greater the chance that the patient's neurological condition at the time of examination may have evolved since the impact.

A history of unconsciousness following the injury indicates that there has been a significant blow. The duration of unconsciousness should be recorded. The patient should be asked about headache and vomiting, about symptoms related to cranial nerve injuries—diplopia, facial numbness, facial weakness, deafness, dysarthria—and about symptoms of weakness or altered sensation in the limbs.

Severe headache and/or vomiting after a head injury are worrying symptoms, and are indications that the patient should be admitted. They may herald an intracranial haematoma or meningitis.

Note whether there has been any bleeding or discharge of fluid from the nose or ears.

Any history of the consumption of alcohol or other drugs should be recorded. The patient's altered state of consciousness may in part be due to alcohol, and evidence of alcohol consumption may be of medico-legal importance. A history of chronic alcohol abuse draws attention to the possibilities of alcohol withdrawal symptoms after admission and of impaired blood coagulation.

If the patient is to be discharged from the Accident Department it is necessary to establish whether there will be adequate supervision at home. If the patient has had a significant injury but is thought not to require admission written instructions should be provided for the next of kin, who should be encouraged to bring the patient back if there is any cause for concern. Absence of suitable supervision at home is an indication for observation in hospital.

- **Has the patient had a head injury?**
- **Always consider the possibility of a head injury in patients with altered consciousness.**
- **Look for signs of trauma.**
- **X-ray the skull.**

The examination

- **The scalp   Vital signs   Conscious level   Cranial nerves   The limbs   The spine   General examination**

In head injury, as in other forms of trauma, it is important to adhere to the standard sequence of **airway**, **breathing**, and **circulation** when carrying out the initial assessment and resuscitation. These priorities must be dealt with appropriately before a more detailed examination is performed.

The scalp

Examine the scalp for evidence of trauma. These signs may be confined to small scalp abrasions or contusions. Scalp lacerations must be carefully explored for fractures and foreign bodies; but this should be delayed until the doctor is prepared to suture the wound, since examination may provoke fresh bleeding. The ear should be drawn forwards so that bruising over the mastoid bone can be seen (Battle's sign), indicating fracture of the petrous bone. Examine the ears with an otoscope for evidence of haemotympanum, which may be found in association with fractures of the petrous bone. Periorbital bruising is evidence of a fracture of the anterior cranial fossa, which may involve the cribriform plate or paranasal air sinuses. Patients with fractures of the base of the anterior fossa or the petrous bone are at risk of developing meningitis. The nose and ears should be inspected for evidence of bleeding or CSF discharge.

Vital signs

The pulse and blood-pressure are recorded and are taken

repeatedly at half-hourly or hourly intervals, depending on the severity of the injury, while the patient remains under observation. A variety of patterns of pulse and blood-pressure is seen, depending on the severity of the injury and the extent of associated injuries.

Commonly, in the unconscious patient, hypertension and tachycardia are the initial findings. Once the airway has been cleared and any injured limbs have been splinted the pulse and blood-pressure may return to normal values. Hypertension with bradycardia implies raised intracranial pressure; but this is by no means always found in patients with an intracranial mass, and, when present, is often a late development. Hypotension is very rarely due to the head injury itself, and should suggest the possibility of blood loss. Hypotension may also be seen in the patient with spinal-cord injury.

Conscious level

Record the patient's state of alertness and conscious level using the Glasgow Coma Scale or its modified form in the case of a child (see Box 8.4, p. 134). The Coma Scale allows conscious level to be recorded in a precise and objective fashion, so that subsequent changes in consciousness can be recognized (see Box 1.3, p. 15). Note that restlessness may be due either to hypoxia or to the brain injury, and that when a previously drowsy, quiet patient becomes restless this may be due either to respiratory deterioration or to a developing intracranial mass.

Cranial nerves

Examine the cranial nerves when appropriate. Detailed examination of each cranial nerve is indicated only if circumstances suggest the possibility of a cranial-nerve injury. Examination of the cranial nerves must not be neglected simply because the patient is not fully conscious. It is quite possible to examine most of the cranial nerves without the patient's co-operation. Injuries of the cranial nerves are discussed in Chapter 6.

Olfactory nerves

The sense of smell can be tested in the conscious patient by occluding one nostril and presenting any strongly scented substance to the other nostril. The patient should indicate whether the scent is apparent, and need not be able to name the substance.

Optic nerves

In the head-injured patient the optic fundi are invariably normal in the hours immediately following the injury. Retinal haemorrhages may be seen in those patients who have collapsed as a result of spontaneous intracranial haemorrhage. It is not desirable to dilate the pupils in order to see the optic fundi, since the pupil's size and reaction to light are an important part of continuing neurological observations.

Visual acuity is measured using either the Snellen chart set at 6 metres (20 feet) from the patient or books of standard print (for example, Jaeger charts). If the patient uses spectacles these should be worn at first one eye and then the other is tested separately.

To examine the visual fields the examiner sits facing the patient and covers one of the patient's eyes with his or her own hand. The patient is then asked to look at the examiner's pupil while an object is brought into the field of vision. A pin-head may be used as the object or, failing that, the examiner's finger. Each quadrant of the field of vision is tested in one eye and then in the other. The patient is asked to indicate when the pin-head is seen, or when a small movement of the examiner's fingertip is recognized. Visual field defects are rarely seen on initial assessment, as they usually follow severe injuries, and require the patient's co-operation.

Cranial nerves 3–6

Record the pupil sizes and their reactions to light. Dilatation of the pupil and an absent light reflex indicate a defect in either the afferent limb or the efferent limb of the light reflex. An afferent pupillary defect is due to injury of the retina or the optic nerve, whereas an efferent pupillary defect is caused by a lesion of the third (oculomotor) cranial nerve or a direct injury of the iris. Injury of the third (oculomotor) nerve may be aused by direct trauma associated with a skull-base fracture, or indirectly as a result of herniation of the temporal lobe through the tentorial hiatus. In the latter case the dilated pupil will be associated with impaired consciousness, whereas in the case of a direct injury of the eye or the nerve alone the patient will be alert, but may have other evidence of injury to the orbit.

By using the consensual reflex it is possible to demonstrate whether unilateral loss of the light reflex is due to an afferent or an efferent defect. In the case of an afferent defect, the pupil will react in response to stimulus to the other eye. In the case of an efferent defect, the pupil of the opposite eye will react in response to a light shone in the abnormal eye. Since the oculomotor nerve is also responsible for the innervation of some extra-ocular muscles and levator palpebrae its injury may be accompanied by a ptosis and ocular palsy.

Examine the eye movements by asking the patient to follow a moving finger. In the uncooperative patient observation alone may reveal impairment of eye movements. However, eye movements can be examined more precisely in the unconscious patient using the oculo-cephalic or 'doll's eye' reflex. As the patient's head is turned from side to side the reflex causes conjugate deviation of the eyes to the opposite side, and so the integrity of the oculomotor and abducent nerves can be established.

Trigeminal nerve
Facial sensation should be tested on either side using a pin. Examine the forehead, cheek, and chin on either side. Subtle degrees of trigeminal sensory impairment may be recognized by testing the corneal reflex with a piece of cotton wool. The corneal reflex can be used to examine trigeminal nerve integrity in the unconscious patient.

Facial nerve
Facial weakness may be due to either an upper or a lower motor lesion. Upper motor-neurone facial weakness may be associated with a hemiparesis, and tends to spare the forehead. The lower motor-neurone lesion involves all the facial muscles. By inflicting a painful stimulus and observing the facial movement in response, it is possible to recognize a facial weakness in the unconscious patient.

Auditory and vestibular nerves

Deafness is not uncommon after head injuries where there has been disruption of the middle-ear apparatus or fractures of the petrous bone.

The simplest technique for detecting deafness is to cover one ear and determine whether the whispered voice can be heard in the other ear. Using a tuning-fork, Rinne's and Weber's tests reveal which ear is deaf and whether the deafness is neural or conductive.

Cranial nerves 9–12

The lower cranial nerves are very infrequently affected in head injuries, and their examination is required only if the patient has post-traumatic dysarthria.

The limbs

Examine the limbs for power and reflexes. Subtle degrees of limb weakness may be missed if the patient is simply asked to 'squeeze my fingers'. A mild hemiparesis can be unmasked by asking the patient to hold out the hands while closing the eyes. The weak arm will drift away from the initial position. In the unconscious patient, observation of the patient's spontaneous movements will reveal asymmetries indicating unilateral weakness. It may be significant that the unconscious patient makes purposeful movements with the left hand in preference to the right.

The spine

Palpate the entire length of the spine for tenderness and examine for bruising. Where there is suspicion of a spinal injury the limbs should be carefully examined for power and reflexes, and a careful sensory examination should be carried out, not neglecting the saddle area.

General examination

If the patient smells of alcohol record this. Finally, a general examination should be carried out, particularly in the unconscious patient, who may be harbouring multiple injuries.

Investigations

Most head-injured patients require minimal investigation. The main consideration in most is whether a skull X-ray should be carried out. Controversy has surrounded the question of who should have skull X-rays. By no means all patients seen in the Accident Department after head injuries require X-rays, and the indications are given in Box 2.2. Essential skull views are the antero-posterior, the lateral, and the Townes view. Interpretation of skull X-rays is discussed in detail in Chapter 5. The main purpose of the skull X-ray is to determine whether the patient requires admission to hospital.

Box 2.2 **Indications for skull X-ray**

- A history of unconsciousness
- Scalp-bruising, haematoma, laceration
- A focal neurological deficit
- An impaired conscious level
- Difficulty in patient-assessment due to age, alcohol, drugs, etc.
- CSF rhinorrhoea or otorrhoea
- Headache, vomiting
- Unconscious, ? head injury

All patients with altered consciousness should have the blood sugar measured by the stick method. Altered consciousness may be due to insulin, oral hypoglycaemic agents, or alcohol.

Other investigations may be indicated by the circumstances of the injury. It should be remembered that injuries of the cervical spine are associated with head injuries when the accident has been a fall or a road-traffic accident. Good-quality X-rays of the cervical spine must include the seventh cervical vertebra on the lateral projection. It may be necessary to pull the shoulders down while the lateral X-ray is taken in order to visualize the lower parts of the cervical spine.

Alcohol levels may be assayed in blood, breath, or saliva. A blood-alcohol level less than 2g/litre makes it likely that altered consciousness is due to the head injury and not to alcohol consumption. It must be emphasized, however, that a high alcohol level cannot be assumed to be the reason for altered consciousness in the injured patient.

Indications for admission to hospital

• Head injury associated with alcohol or drug ingestion

The unconscious or multiply-injured patient clearly requires admission. The conscious patient may require admission either because there is a scalp or skull injury which is unsuitable for outpatient treatment or because there are reasons to believe that the injury may be attended by delayed complications. The latter group of patients are admitted for observation and symptomatic relief.

The main source of anxiety in the case of the patient with a relatively mild primary injury is the possibility of extradural haematoma. In adult patients 80 per cent of extradural haematomas are associated with a skull fracture—recognized either clinically or radiologically. In children 40 per cent of extradural haematomas occur without radiological evidence of a fracture. The presence of a skull fracture is, therefore, the most important risk factor in determining who is in danger of developing this potentially lethal complication. The absence of a fracture is less reassuring in children, and the indications for admission have to be broader.

The patient with a skull fracture who is not fully conscious has been shown to have as much as a 25 per cent chance of having an intracranial haematoma of some sort.

In contrast, the conscious patient with no skull fracture has only a 1 in 6000 chance of developing an intracranial haematoma. Box 2.3 describes the risks of intracranial haematoma in different groups of patients.

In adults, a history of unconsciousness following the injury is not in itself an indication for admission, since it is associated with a very low incidence of intracranial haema-

Box 2.3 **Risk of intracranial haematoma after head injury**

		Risk of intracranial haematoma
Orientated	No skull fracture	1 in 6000
Disorientated	No skull fracture	1 in 120
Orientated	Skull fracture	1 in 30
Disorientated	Skull fracture	1 in 4

toma. In children, however, it is prudent to observe the patient who has had an injury severe enough to cause loss of consciousness, partly because the absence of a skull fracture is a less reliable indication of the risk of intracranial haematoma, and partly because recognition of deterioration in the child is more difficult than in the adult. Even in good health the young child may be difficult to rouse after the accustomed bedtime, and this tendency is more pronounced when the child is overwrought and exhausted after the drama of injury and hospital attendance.

Severe headache and vomiting may be symptoms of an intracranial haematoma in the patient who is fully conscious and exhibits no focal neurological deficit.

The patient with CSF rhinorrhoea or otorrhoea should be admitted until the discharge has ceased or the fistula has been repaired.

Extensive scalp lacerations should be repaired under general anaesthetic, and may be associated with significant blood loss.

The patient who has had a fit following injury may have further post-traumatic fits, and should be admitted for observation. There is a very small increased incidence of intracranial haematoma in association with post-traumatic fits.

Head injury associated with alcohol or drug ingestion

There is a strong association between alcohol and head injury, and the patient's clinical condition may be due to a combination of alcohol intoxication and head injury. In the case of a drowsy head-injured patient who has had a surfeit

Box 2.4 **Indications for admission**

- Altered conscious level
- Post-traumatic epileptic fit
- Focal neurological deficit
- Clinical or radiological evidence of skull fracture
- Severe headache or vomiting
- CSF rhinorrhoea/otorrhoea
- Extensive scalp laceration
- Inadequate supervision at home
- Child with history of unconsciousness

of alcohol it is not possible to predict the contribution made to the altered conscious state by alcohol. One must always assume that the patient's impaired conscious level is due to head injury, and investigate or observe the patient appropriately.

As has been mentioned, the skull X-ray plays an important part in the decision to admit the head-injured patient to hospital. Very often the X-rays have to be interpreted by a relatively inexperienced doctor at hours when more experienced advice is not immediately available. A reliable history may not always be obtainable, and social circumstances may raise doubts as to how well the patient will be observed at home. The foregoing criteria for admission are only guidelines, and the doctor on the spot must always act on the side of caution if there is any doubt about the significance of the injury.

Having decided that the patient requires admission, the next step is to ensure that any subsequent neurological deterioration is recognized early and acted upon.

Neurological observation

In most instances, the purpose of admitting the head-injured patient is to enable potential complications to be recognized at an early and treatable stage. To this end, observations should be directed towards recognizing neurological deterioration and evidence of a developing intracranial haematoma or other secondary causes of neurological impairment. Conscious level is also assessed at hourly intervals in the terms of the Glasgow Coma Scale. It is convenient to chart all the observations on a single neurological observation chart (Fig. 2.1). It is important to make sure that the medical and nursing staff understand the terms of the Coma Scale in order to avoid spurious apparent changes in conscious level.

Pulse-rate, blood-pressure, temperature, and respiratory rate should be recorded at hourly intervals. Bradycardia and hypertension are associated with rising intracranial pressure. The size of the pupils and their reaction to light are also recorded hourly. Dilatation of one pupil or a sluggish or absent response to light is an ominous sign, indicating a developing mass on the same side as the affected pupil. These signs develop in the late stages of rising intracranial pressure.

The patient with a moderate concussional head injury will usually tend to lie quietly with the eyes closed unless disturbed. If the patient begins to become restless, exhibiting purposeless activity, such as pulling at the bedclothes or making ineffectual efforts to get over the cot-sides, this represents a deterioration in conscious level. On no account should restless head-injured patients be sedated. This behaviour may herald the development of an intracranial haematoma, and should be investigated appropriately. In the absence of an operable intracranial lesion these patients can usually be contained by cot-sides on the bed and nursing supervision.

Never sedate the restless head-injured patient.

If it is clear after 12 to 24 hours that the patient is steadily improving the frequency of the recordings may be reduced. Most head-injured patients will need observation for approximately 24 hours, by which time there is little likelihood of delayed deterioration, and the patient may be discharged as soon as symptoms such as headache or vomiting allow.

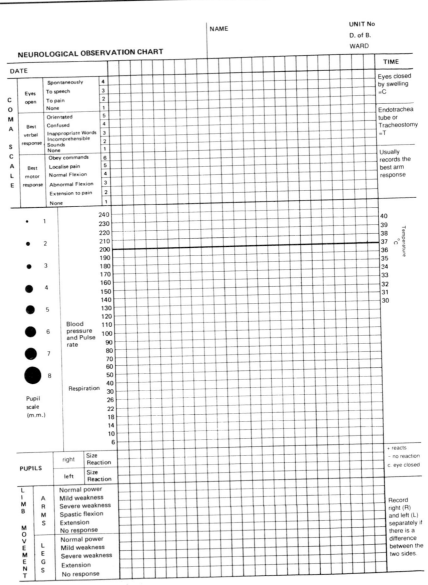

Fig. 2.1 • A neurological observation chart (Aberdeen hospitals CNS observation chart).

Patients should be discharged to the care of a responsible adult who has been given advice about simple head-injury observation and when to seek further medical attention. Relatives should not be asked to carry out formal hourly observations—particularly through the night. If this level of observation is really required the patient should be admitted to hospital rather than being sent home. Friends or relatives should be advised to bring the patient back to hospital if there is severe headache, persistent vomiting, confusion, or drowsiness. The patient should be advised to report any discharge of dilute fluid from the nose or ears.

Box 2.5   Head-injury instructions

Seek further medical advice in the event of:
- Severe headache
- Frequent vomiting
- Discharge of fluid from nose or ears
- Confusion or inappropriate drowsiness

Relief of symptoms

Analgesics are required for headache, but strong opioid analgesics should be avoided, particularly in the drowsy or confused patient. Simple oral analgesics such as paracetamol or codeine phosphate are suitable for relatively minor pain. Non-steroidal anti-inflammatory agents such as diclofenac are also effective, and the latter can be administered orally, intramuscularly, or in suppository form. The conscious patient with more severe pain must be given effective analgesia, and this can be achieved using reversible opioids such as morphine or papaveritum (omnopon) intravenously, titrated to the patient's response while concern about possible intracranial complications persists. Local anaesthetic blocks may be used in some instances for relief of limb pain if narcotic analgesics are to be avoided; such blocks are most effective in the patient with a head injury complicated by a solitary limb injury.

Nausea and vomiting can be controlled with any of the standard antiemetic agents.

Outpatient review

Of the patients seen in Accident and Emergency Departments and either discharged or admitted for observation only a small number should be reviewed, and most of these should be seen in the relevant specialist departments. Patients with cranial nerve injuries must be reviewed in Neurosurgery, ENT, or Ophthalmology clinics as appropriate. Patients with post-traumatic epilepsy, if not already under the care of a neurosurgeon, should be reviewed in a Neurosurgical Clinic. Post-concussional symptoms are dealt with in most instances by General Practitioners, and only occasionally require specialist referral.

Patients with uncomplicated head injuries do not require routine review in the Accident and Emergency Department.

Further reading

Bickerstaff E. R. (1980). *Neurological examination in clinical practice.* Blackwell Scientific Publications, Oxford.

Jennett, Bryan and Teasdale, Graham (1981). *Management of head injuries.* F. A. Davis Co., Philadelphia.

Tyson, G. W. (1987). *Head injury management for providers of emergency care.* Williams and Wilkins, Baltimore.

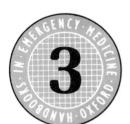

Chapter 3

Resuscitation

Key points in resuscitation

1 Resuscitation of the head-injured patient is the responsibility of the A&E Department, and on no account should a patient be transferred to a specialist unit before resuscitation is complete and the patient stabilized. Hypotension and hypoxia on arrival at Neurosurgery are associated with very high mortality rates. Patients should not be removed from the resuscitation room (for example, for X-rays) until resuscitation is complete: this may necessitate the use of portable X-ray equipment.

2 Until it is proved otherwise patients should be assumed to have associated cervical-spine injuries, and up to that point the neck should be immobilized with a rigid collar or between sandbags, and a senior member of the team should be in charge of the head and neck whenever a patient is moved.

3 Opioid analgesics and benzodiazepines should be administered with great care, and only when facilities to reverse their effects and to ventilate the patient are available, because of their respiratory-depressant action.

4 Gaining control of the airway and ventilation is vital in controlling intracranial pressure and hypoxia, and failure in this can render any direct management of the head injury futile: the A&E doctor should never hesitate to ventilate in advance of a neurosurgical opinion if respiration is inadequate.

5 When deciding to use positive-pressure ventilation care must be taken to exclude or to treat a pneumothorax first.

6 Endotracheal intubation and controlled ventilation should be instituted by an anaesthetist or a doctor experienced in anaesthetic technique, with an assistant applying pressure to the cricoid cartilage to prevent regurgitation of gastric contents.

7 $PaCO_2$ should be maintained between 3.5 and 4.0 kPa.

8 A CT scan is mandatory in the patient whose conscious level is deteriorating; in the patient who remains unconscious after resuscitation, with a Glasgow Coma Score of 8 or less; and in the patient with a skull fracture who is not fully conscious.

9 Anaesthetic techniques used for the treatment of other injuries must avoid exacerbating raised intracranial pressure.

10 Pain causes increased intracranial pressure in the head-injured, but opioid analgesics, including codeine, depress consciousness and respiration even in small doses, and so if used they should be given in small intravenous aliquots under close observation.

Priorities in resuscitation

• **Cervical spine**

Resuscitation of the head-injured patient is the responsibility of the staff in the Accident and Emergency Department, and the outcome of the injury depends crucially on the effectiveness of this early stage in the patient's treatment. It cannot be stressed too often that general resuscitation must precede all other considerations.

The management of severe head injuries is governed by the same principles as that of other forms of trauma— **Airway, Breathing, and Circulation**, in that order of priority. It is easy to be distracted by the apparent severity of the head injury, especially, for example, when there is a major compound injury; but the successful management of the head injury depends first and foremost on the effectiveness of the general resuscitation. On no account should the head-injured patient be transferred to a specialist unit before resuscitative measures have been completed and the patient's condition has been stabilized.

> **Head-injury resuscitation is the responsibility of the doctor in the Accident and Emergency Department.**

A study in Glasgow in 1981 by Gentleman and Jennett illustrated the influence of extracranial injuries on the outcome after head injury. Patients with hypotension and/or hypoxia were compared with those with neither complication. Patients who were hypotensive on arrival in the Neurosurgical Unit had a mortality rate of 75 per cent, and those who were hypoxic a mortality rate of 59 per cent. There were no survivors in the group who had been both hypotensive and hypoxic. This was compared with a 34 per cent mortality in those patients who had suffered neither insult. A study by Koni and Mendelow in 1984 showed similarly unfavourable results when the quality of outcome in surviving patients was related to the occurrence of hypotension and hypoxia.

Clinical assessment, resuscitation, and investigation must

be conducted simultaneously in the resuscitation room. Appropriate early investigations are those that will contribute directly to the process of resuscitation. In general the patient should not be moved from the resuscitation room (for instance, for the purpose of X-rays) until resuscitation is complete. This may require X-rays of the chest, cervical spine, or pelvis to be performed using portable equipment. X-rays of minor limb injuries or obvious fractures are not required until resuscitation has been completed.

Box 3.1 Priorities in resuscitation

- Stabilize cervical spine
- Airway
- Breathing
- Circulation
- Neurological assessment

Cervical spine

Until it is proved otherwise, head-injured patients arriving in the Accident Department should be assumed to have an associated spinal injury. Until this has been assessed clinically and radiologically the neck should be immobilized, either with a rigid collar or, in the case of the deeply unconscious patient, between sandbags. Care must be exercised when moving the patient (for instance, from the ambulance trolley to the Accident and Emergency trolley). A senior member of the team should be in charge of the head and neck whenever it is necessary to lift the patient from one surface to another.

Airway and breathing

- **Central respiratory impairment   Peripheral respiratory impairment   Airway management   Intubation and ventilation**

Respiratory insufficiency commonly accompanies head injury, and constitutes the most important cause of avoidable morbidity and mortality. Respiratory insufficiency is due either to **central factors** or to **peripheral factors**.

Central respiratory impairment

The unconscious patient readily obstructs the upper airway because of the tendency of the tongue to fall back and occlude the oropharynx. Loss of the protective airway reflexes exposes the patient to the risk of vomiting and aspirating gastric contents. Abnormal patterns of respiration are seen in the unconscious head-injured patient; but respiratory depression directly due to the brain injury itself is rare, except as a terminal event. Central depression of respiration is more commonly due to the effects of alcohol, drugs, or epileptic fits. Opioid analgesics and benzodiazepines are potent respiratory depressants in the head-injured patient, and should be administered with great care, and only when facilities are available to reverse their effects and to ventilate the patient. Epileptic fits, due to either the primary brain injury, hypoxia, or a known previous epileptic condition, will cause respiratory insufficiency. Most fits are self-limiting; but prolonged fits (status epilepticus) or recurrent fits require treatment, partly because of respiratory considerations. All the drugs used to treat status epilepticus can cause respiratory depression, and must be used with appropriate caution.

Box 3.2   **Causes of respiratory impairment**

Central causes
- Drugs
- Brain-stem injury

Peripheral causes
- Airway obstruction
- Aspiration of blood/vomit
- Chest trauma
- Adult respiratory distress syndrome
- Pulmonary oedema

Peripheral respiratory impairment

Upper airway obstruction may be caused by blood, teeth, or

dentures, or by fractures of the facial skeleton. Fractures of the facial skeleton cause respiratory impairment either because of severe associated haemorrhage or because the posterior displacement of the face itself occludes the oropharynx. The severe impacted facial fracture is recognized by a 'dish-faced' deformity and by bilateral periorbital haematomas. Fractures of the mandible may also be associated with respiratory obstruction, particularly if bilateral fractures exist and the patient is lying horizontally in the supine position.

Chest and head injuries commonly coexist in the same patient. Inspection will reveal contusions of the chest wall, asymmetrical expansion, and paradoxical movement. Surgical emphysema indicates the presence of a pneumothorax. An early chest X-ray is an essential part of the process of resuscitation. The chest X-ray may show rib fractures, pulmonary contusion, and pneumothorax. The latter may not be obvious on the supine chest X-ray, which should be repeated if there is clinical evidence of respiratory impairment. Similarly, pulmonary contusion may not be obvious on an early X-ray, and after the passage of an hour or two a further X-ray can show an alarming change in a contused lung.

'Neurogenic' pulmonary oedema sometimes occurs as a result of severe brain injuries, and is often resistant to diuretic therapy. Since early correction of respiratory impairment is so critically important it is not sufficient to treat pulmonary oedema with diuretics alone, and positive-pressure ventilation is essential.

Adult respiratory distress syndrome, fat embolus, and chest infection are complications which present after the period of initial resuscitation, and are discussed in Chapter 4.

Impaired ventilation has a very important bearing on the outcome of the head injury. Firstly, the already injured brain can ill tolerate the additional insult of hypoxia, and the conscious level may deteriorate dramatically as a result. Secondly, the arterial $PaCO_2$ has an important direct effect on intracranial pressure. Cerebral arterioles dilate in response to a rise in $PaCO_2$, with a consequent increase in cerebral blood-flow and intracranial blood-volume, and intracranial pressure is elevated. Since intracranial pressure may already be critically elevated by brain swelling or intracranial haemorrhage, every effort must be made to avoid any further exacerbation. These effects are immediate and require urgent action. Hence, gaining control of the airway and ventilation is absolutely vital. Failure to do so renders any effort directed towards direct management of the head injury futile. This is so important that **the doctor in the Accident and Emergency Department should never be deterred from proceeding to ventilate the patient in advance of a neurosurgical opinion if the patient's respiration is inadequate.**

Airway management

Management of the airway begins with the removal of any upper-airway obstruction. This is done under direct vision with the aid of a laryngoscope, McGill forceps, and a Yankauer sucker. The mouth and pharynx must be cleared of teeth, blood, and vomit. The airway should then be kept patent by preventing obstruction by the tongue. The examiner's fingers are placed behind the angles of the mandibles and the mandible is drawn forwards—the 'jaw thrust' manoeuvre. A Guedel oral airway should be inserted. The patient who will not tolerate an oral airway should be nursed in the lateral ('recovery') position once resuscitation is complete. Bleeding from facial fractures can be torrential, and may in its own right make endotracheal intubation necessary in order to protect the airway.

Intubation and ventilation

The head-injured patient who has inadequate respiration requires intubation and positive-pressure ventilation as a matter of priority. Ventilation is indicated for the reasons listed in Box 3.3. It may be impossible to maintain a clear upper airway simply by using an oral airway. Chest-wall or pulmonary injury may result in impaired gas-exchange, with inadequate PaO_2 and elevated $PaCO_2$ when the patient is breathing spontaneously. When deciding to use positive-pressure ventilation care must be taken to exclude a pneumothorax, or to treat it by tube thoracostomy if one is present. Flail segments should be obvious on direct inspection, but a pneumothorax may not be so easily recognized, and positive-pressure ventilation will exacerbate the problem if the pneumothorax is not drained. When a significant chest injury is found it is likely that, sooner or later, respiratory efficiency will deteriorate, and the patient's neurological condition with it. The PaO_2 should not be allowed to fall below 10.5 kPa (80 mm Hg).

> **The head-injured patient who is not breathing effectively requires urgent ventilation.**

If endotracheal intubation and controlled ventilation are indicated, these procedures should be carried out by an anaesthetist or a doctor fully experienced in anaesthetic technique, using an induction agent such as thiopentone, propofol, or etomidate and a short-acting paralysing agent.

Box 3.3 **Indications for ventilation**

- Upper-airway protection —Obstruction by tongue
  —Facial injuries
- Poor respiratory effort —Central respiratory depression
  —Drugs, such as analgesics anticonvulsants
- Aspiration of gastric contents
- Pulmonary oedema
- Chest injury —Multiple fractured ribs
  —Flail chest
  —Pulmonary contusion
- A suspected intracranial mass
- Transporting a severely injured patient
- Status epilepticus

During intubation an assistant should apply pressure to the cricoid cartilage (Sellick's manoeuvre) in order to prevent regurgitation of gastric contents. The 'crash' intubation by an inexperienced doctor in a struggling patient exacerbates an already raised intracranial pressure, and may be extremely damaging.

Box 3.4 Induction of anaesthesia for intubation and controlled ventilation

Induction agent	Thiopentone sodium	100–150 mg i.v. over 10–15 sec. 4–8 mg/kg in child
	Propofol	2.0–2.5 mg/kg i.v. 20–40 mg every 10 sec.
	Etomidate	300 micrograms/kg i.v. slow injection until patient anaesthetized
Paralysing agent	Suxamethonium chloride	0.6 mg/kg
	Atracurium	0.3–0.6 mg/kg

Chest X-rays and arterial blood-gas readings must be taken again once the patient has been intubated and controlled ventilation has been established.

Box 3.5 Early investigations

- Chest X-ray
- Arterial blood gases
- X-ray of cervical spine
- X-ray of pelvis
- Cross-matching of blood
- Skull X-rays
- Blood alcohol

Arterial blood gases should be analysed regularly during resuscitation. Correction of hypoxia may make a dramatic difference to the conscious level. Hypoxia may not be clinically obvious in the young, previously fit patient, and may only be revealed by blood-gas analysis.

Having decided to ventilate the patient it is important to ensure that paralysis and sedation are maintained. This is achieved by the use of a sedative agent and a long-acting neuromuscular blocking agent given intermittently or by continuous infusion. If the patient is allowed to become 'light' and struggles against the ventilator intracranial pressure will be increased.

Box 3.6 **Drugs used for paralysis and sedation of the ventilated adult patient**

Sedation	• Papaveretum (omnopon)	i.v. infusion 2–5 mg/hour
	• Phenoperidine	i.v. infusion 1 mg/hour
	• Alfentanil	i.v. infusion 2–4 mg/hour
	• Propofol	i.v. infusion 100–200 micrograms/kg/min.
Paralysis	• Atracurium	i.v. infusion 300–600 micrograms/kg/hour
	• Pancuronium bromide	i.v. injection 60 micrograms/kg/1–2 hours

---

An oxygen-saturation monitor is a most useful aid in the care of the head-injured patient once a steady state has been reached, particularly when it is necessary to transfer the patient to the X-ray department or to another hospital. It cannot however measure oxygen saturation accurately in the shocked patient. After the phase of initial resuscitation respiratory impairment remains a common cause of neurological deterioration.

Intermittent positive-pressure ventilation not only ensures

that respiration is supported, but can be used to reduce the intracranial pressure by lowering the $PaCO_2$. The $PaCO_2$ should be maintained between 3.5 and 4.0 kPa. $PaCO_2$ below 3 kPa causes a degree of cerebral vasoconstriction which may cause cerebral ischaemia. It is particularly important to control the $PaCO_2$ in the case of the deteriorating patient who is suspected of harbouring an intracranial haematoma. Controlled ventilation reduces the intracranial pressure and allows time to transfer the patient, arrange the CT scan, or open the operating theatre. Ventilation as part of the subsequent management of the severe brain injury is discussed in Chapter 4.

In general, the more extensive the injuries in the multiply injured patient the greater the indication for intubation and ventilation.

Circulation and blood volume

The physiological mechanism of cerebrovascular autoregulation ensures that cerebral blood-flow remains constant despite fluctuations in systemic blood-pressure. This mechanism is impaired after head injuries, and cerebral perfusion is at the mercy of the systemic blood-pressure. Consequently, blood loss and hypotension have a serious impact on cerebral perfusion. Moreover, cerebral perfusion may already be compromised by elevated intracranial pressure. As far as the head injury is concerned, then, it is an urgent matter to recognize circulatory impairment due to blood loss or reduced cardiac output.

The physiological response to raised intracranial pressure includes a rise in blood-pressure and a slowing of pulse-rate (the 'Cushing reflex'). This may have the effect of masking shock, and it is necessary to recognize that 'shock' in the head-injured patient has different parameters from shock in other individuals. If the patient with a severe head injury has a systolic blood-pressure of 100–110mm Hg and a pulse-rate of 100/min. it is likely that there is concealed extracranial haemorrhage.

It is essential that blood volume is restored and haemorrhage is arrested before consideration is given to any form of neurosurgical intervention. There is no value in operative neurosurgical intervention if the brain is not being perfused.

Blood loss and hypotension further exacerbate impaired cerebral perfusion.

Serious blood loss from the head injury alone is uncommon, except in the case of small children, and other sources should be sought. Serious head injuries are commonly associated with injuries of the chest, abdomen, pelvis, and limbs, and the treatment of continuing haemorrhage from one of these sources takes priority over cranial surgery and neurological investigations such as CT scan. It may be appropriate, for instance, to take the patient to the operating theatre for a splenectomy first, and, having gained control of the blood loss, then turn one's attention to the neurological problem.

Head-down tilting, for instance, for the purpose of inserting a central venous catheter, should be avoided, since this leads to a further rise in intracranial pressure, and can lead to neurological deterioration.

Nasogastric intubation and urinary catheterization

Nasogastric intubation in the unconscious patient may be desirable in certain circumstances, such as in the case of associated abdominal injuries or in the patient who is thought to have a full stomach. There are hazards in passing a nasogastric tube, however. The procedure may induce retching or vomiting, with potential ill effects on the head injury through raising the intracranial pressure. Great care should be exercised in passing a nasogastric tube in the patient with major skull-base fractures, as there is a risk that the tube will pass through the fracture into the cranial cavity. In such cases, orogastric intubation should be performed.

Catheterization of the bladder may be desirable in the case of severe multiple injuries with hypotension; but it is not necessary in the management of the patient who has only sustained a head injury. The unconscious patient will void urine perfectly satisfactorily, and, in the male, a urinary sheath will often suffice. The unconscious female patient will require a urinary catheter.

Other injuries

Cervical spine fractures are commonly associated with head injuries, and in the early period after admission there is a considerable risk that further damage may be inflicted during intubation and transfer from trolley to X-ray couch and bed. Throughout the period of resuscitation the possibility of a cervical spine injury should be remembered, and the head and neck should be controlled whenever the patient is moved. The conscious patient will complain of neck pain in the presence of a spinal injury; but the unconscious patient must be treated as if the cervical spine has been injured until it is proved otherwise. A full-length lateral X-ray of the cervical spine, and an antero-posterior view showing the odontoid process are required. If a cervical fracture or sub-luxation is suspected the neck should be splinted in a rigid collar; but care must be taken to ensure that this is not applied so tightly that cerebral venous return is obstructed.

Other injuries may demand early attention; but it is necessary at this stage, having stabilized respiration and blood volume, to assess the patient's neurological condition.

Neurological assessment

• Indications for CT scan

The most important aspect of the neurological assessment is to determine whether and how the patient's conscious level is changing. The severity of the initial brain injury is reflected by the patient's conscious level at the time of injury and after resuscitation. The management of this primary brain injury amounts to providing a suitable physiological environment in which to enable spontaneous recovery to take place. A minority of patients will have a progressive neurological condition due to intracranial haemorrhage, and this is recognized by a deterioration in conscious level following the initial impact.

Conscious level may be affected by systemic factors described above (hypotension, hypoxia), and it is necessary to record the patient's conscious level after resuscitation has been affected. Regular conscious level recordings are then carried out along with measurements of pulse-rate, blood-pressure, respiratory rate, and temperature. Any deterioration in conscious level from this point is an indication of some secondary brain injury, as was outlined in Chapter 4.

As part of the neurological examination, the scalp should be carefully examined for external evidence of injury. Penetrating head injuries may be hidden by hair unless the scalp is closely inspected. Bruising over the mastoid process and periorbital haematomas are noted as evidence of skull-base injury. Examine the ears and nose for evidence of cerebro-spinal fluid leakage. The pupil size and responsiveness to light are recorded, as are focal neurological deficits. Limb weakness may only be recognized by observing the patient's spontaneous movements or responses to painful stimuli.

Box 3.7 Neurological assessment

- Conscious level (Glasgow Coma Scale)
- Pupil size and light reflex
- Scalp injuries
- CSF otorrhoea/rhinorrhoea
- Limb weakness

At this stage skull X-rays should be carried out, since the presence of a skull fracture is an important risk factor in the recognition of extradural haematoma.

Indications for CT scan

Following resuscitation and the establishment of a neurological baseline, consideration should be given to whether further neurological investigations are required. The criteria for CT scanning are detailed in Box 3.8, but it must be emphasized that a CT scan is mandatory in the patient whose conscious level is deteriorating and in the patient who remains unconscious after resuscitation, with a Glasgow Coma Score of 8 or less. A scan is also indicated in the patient with a skull fracture who is not fully conscious, since this combination of factors is associated with a 25 per cent incidence of intracranial haematoma of some sort on CT scan.

Box 3.8   Criteria for CT scan

- Patient remains unconscious after resuscitation (GCS ≤8)
- Patient with depressed conscious level and skull fracture
- Patient with depressed conscious level and focal deficit
- Patient with skull fracture and focal deficit
- Patient with deteriorating conscious level
- Patient with head injury who requires ventilation
- Patient with head injury who requires general anaesthetic for orthopaedic surgery

---

If it is necessary to ventilate the patient for any reason it is no longer possible to monitor conscious level, and a CT scan is necessary in order to exclude an operable intracranial haematoma. A scan is also indicated if it is necessary to anaesthetize the patient for long orthopaedic procedures during which no neurological observations are possible.

After resuscitation and the initial neurological assessment it may be necessary to proceed to surgical treatment of other injuries. Compound fractures and abdominal injuries often require early treatment, and it is well established that major limb fractures are best treated and stabilized early. Great care must be taken to avoid exacerbating the brain injury during this period. Inappropriate anaesthetic technique causing hypoxia, hypercapnia, or raised intracranial pressure together with hypotension can be responsible for further neurological damage. The patient should be cared for by an experienced anaesthetist.

> **Anaesthetic technique must avoid exacerbating raised intracranial pressure.**

Analgesia

The choice of analgesic for the multiply injured patient often causes anxiety. The control of pain is important not only for humanitarian reasons but also because pain causes increased intracranial pressure in the head-injured patient. Opioid analgesics, including codeine, cause depression of consciousness and respiration, and may do so in small doses in the head-injured patient. If they are used they should be administered in small intravenous aliquots, and the patient must be closely observed. The choice of analgesic techniques is discussed in Chapter 2 ('Relief of symptoms').

The management of a patient whose conscious level is deteriorating is discussed in the next chapter.

Further reading

Frost, E. (1977). Respiratory problems associated with head trauma. *Neurosurgery*, **1**, 300–5, 1977.

Jennett, Bryan, and Teasdale, Graham (1981). *Management of head injuries* (chapter 9). F. A. Davis Co., Philadelphia.

Miller, J. D. (1978). Early insults to the injured brain. *Journal of the American Medical Association*, **240**, 439–42.

Gentleman, D., and Jennett, B. (1981). Hazards of inter-hospital transfer of comatose head-injured patients. *Lancet*, **2**, 853–5.

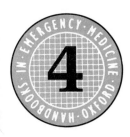

Chapter 4

Neurological
deterioration

Key points in neurological deterioration

1 A very large part of the time and effort spent in the care of head-injured patients is applied to recognizing secondary brain injury.

2 After general resuscitation simple remediable causes of deterioration should be excluded before considering transfer to a Neurosurgical Unit and CT scanning.

3 The commonest of these causes is impaired respiration—hypoxia, or CO_2 retention causing increased intracranial pressure.

4 Impaired respiration is most frequently caused by facial injuries, usually leading to haemorrhage and aspiration of blood, and chest injuries leading to physical difficulties in respiration, and may be delayed in onset until after the early stages of assessment, being eventually precipitated by exhaustion: intubation and ventilation should be considered at an early stage.

5 Once patients have been ventilated a CT scan should be carried out, and transfer to a Neurosurgical Unit should take place, as clinical monitoring of the neurological condition is no longer possible.

6 If an epileptic fit persists for more than 2–3 minutes it should be arrested with diazepam or chlormethiazole; but these should only be used when facilities are available to ventilate the patient in the event of respiratory arrest, because of their respiratory-depressant effects.

7 Where, because of unconsciousness or multiple injuries, anticonvulsants have to be given parenterally to control recurrences of fitting, only phenytoin, sodium valproate, and phenobarbitone can regularly be used: sodium valproate should not be used in women of child-bearing age, because of its teratogenicity, and patients should have blood-pressure and ECG monitoring when phenytoin is administered, because it can cause cardiac arrhythmias and hypotension.

8 Intracranial haematoma should be treated operatively, normally in a Neurosurgical Unit, and where possible after a CT scan. Intracranial pressure can be temporarily reduced (1–2 hours) by intravenous diuretics such as mannitol or fusemide (not to be given to hypovolaemic patients) to facilitate investigations or treatment.

9 The deteriorating patient with an intracranial haematoma should be anaesthetized, paralysed, and ventilated—this is essential for long-distance inter-hospital transfer.

10 An extradural haematoma cannot be treated through a burr-hole: ideally a craniotomy is required, or failing that a burr-hole extended to form a craniectomy.

The effect and outcome of a head injury depends principally on the severity of the initial impact and the extent of the damage thereby caused to the brain. This is the **primary brain injury**, the clinical results of which may range from a brief period of unconsciousness on the one hand to prolonged coma on the other. The pathological effects of the primary injury are discussed in Chapter 1. The clinical effect of the primary brain injury is recognized by the patient's conscious level and the presence and severity of neurological deficits immediately after the impact. If, for example, the patient is capable of speaking after the head injury it is clear that the initial damage to the brain has been relatively slight, and one would expect such a patient to survive the injury if appropriately cared for. The Glasgow School of Neurosurgery has coined the term '**patients who talk and die**' to highlight the fact that the patient who is capable of talking after the injury is expected to survive unless some secondary and avoidable injury is allowed to develop unchecked. On the other hand, the patient who is only extending the limbs in response to a painful stimulus, and whose pupils fail to react to light in the immediate aftermath of the injury has suffered a severe primary injury of the brain, from which complete recovery is much less likely.

Surgical treatment of the primary injury is directed mainly at the repair of scalp and skull injuries and penetrating injuries of the brain. Treatment of the primary brain injury is supportive—the care of the unconscious patient and the prevention of further damage.

Whether the head injury is apparently minor or very severe a number of factors may complicate the injury and cause further insult to the established brain injury. This **secondary brain injury** can be anticipated and avoided or recognized and treated. The secondary injury may further exacerbate a severe primary injury, in which case treatment of the cause of deterioration is expected to restore the patient only to the state determined by the primary injury. In some instances, however, the secondary injury may complicate a relatively minor primary injury which, in itself, poses little threat to the patient. In this case, there is a danger that a patient with a relatively minor injury might die or be disabled by entirely avoidable or treatable factors.

A very large part, therefore, of the effort and time spent in the care of head-injured patients is applied to the task of recognizing the potential secondary brain injury.

The prevention of secondary brain damage depends firstly on recognizing the risk factors for the various complications of head injury described below and secondly on ensuring that deterioration is recognized when it does occur. This, in turn, depends on the correct selection of patients for admission and on the effectiveness of head-injury observations.

Causes of deteriorating conscious level

A number of factors may cause deterioration in conscious level following a head injury. All act directly or indirectly by impairing either cerebral perfusion or the delivery of oxygen to the brain. Intracranial haemorrhage is a well-known com-

---

Box 4.1 Causes of deteriorating conscious level

- **Respiratory impairment** —hypoxia
  —hypercapnia
- **Hypovolaemia** —blood loss
  —reduced cardiac output
- **Obstructed cerebral** —head-down tilt
  venous return —forcible intubation
  —cervical collars
- **Fits**
- **Intracranial haematoma** —extradural haematoma
  —subdural haematoma
  —intracerebral haematoma
- **Fluid overload** —hyponatraemia
- **Drugs** —analgesics
  —sedatives

plication of head injury, causing secondary deterioration; but before jumping to the conclusion that the patient requires immediate transfer and CT scanning it is advisable first to investigate the more immediately remediable causes of deterioration. Indeed, if these systemic complications are not treated promptly the ensuing secondary brain damage may render the question of operative neurosurgical intervention academic. This means that the doctor in the Accident and Emergency Department or the isolated District General Hospital must resist the urge to transfer the deteriorating head-injured patient to a Neurosurgical Unit until general resuscitative measures have been carried out and simply remediable causes of deterioration have been excluded.

Respiratory complications

Impaired respiration is the commonest cause of deteriorating conscious level in the head-injured patient. The injured brain is exquisitely sensitive to **hypoxia**, and the resulting deterioration in conscious level itself will lead to failure to maintain a clear airway and a vicious circle of respiratory impairment.

   CO_2 retention causes cerebral vasodilatation, with a consequent rise in intracranial pressure. Added to an already raised pressure due to swelling of the injured brain, the effect of CO_2 retention may be to cause serious deterioration in conscious level. This effect of impaired respiration is immediate, and requires a rapid response.

   It is possible to anticipate delayed respiratory impairment when the initial assessment of the patient is carried out. The chief culprits in the early stages after injury are facial and chest injuries. The former can cause upper-airway obstruction when there is posterior displacement of the facial skeleton, but more frequently result in haemorrhage and aspiration of blood. Chest injuries may result in respiratory impairment as a result of pain that inhibits chest expansion, pulmonary contusion, pneumothorax, or flail-chest deformity. In the early stages of assessment the patient may appear to cope with these injuries and maintain reasonable respiratory efficiency. Deterioration may be prevented by the use of oxygen by face-mask, appropriate analgesia, and insertion of an intercostal chest drain where indicated. However, as exhaustion supervenes respiratory efforts decrease. It is preferable to anticipate this development; and in the presence of such injuries one should seriously consider paralysing, intubating, and ventilating the patient at an early stage.

Early chest X-ray appearances can be deceptively normal; but after as little as one hour there can be dramatic changes, with the appearance of pneumothorax or contusional changes. Hypoxia and hypercapnia are often underestimated, and are difficult to detect clinically. In the event of a deterioration in conscious level exclude upper-airway obstruction before going on to repeat the chest X-ray and arterial blood-gas analysis.

Check arterial blood gases.

Once the cause of respiratory impairment has been identified simple measures, such as chest physiotherapy and oxygen by face-mask or the insertion of a chest drain may be adequate to correct the patient's arterial blood gases; but, if not, early consideration should be given to artificial ventilation. The head-injured patient who is not breathing effectively must be ventilated as a matter of priority. This is nowhere more vital than when it is proposed to transfer the patient to another hospital. The decision to paralyse and ventilate a head-injured patient in respiratory difficulties should certainly not be postponed until a neurosurgical opinion has been obtained.

The head-injured patient who is not breathing effectively must be ventilated.

Once a patient has been paralysed and ventilated a CT scan should be performed, if this has not already been done, in order to identify any possible intracranial haematoma, since further clinical monitoring of the neurological condition is no longer possible. Thereafter, the only means of following the progress of the head injury in these patients is to monitor the intracranial pressure. These requirements make it necessary for all such patients to be admitted to a Neurosurgical Unit.

Delayed neurological deterioration may occur after an interval of days or weeks as a result of respiratory complications. Since this presents, in many instances, at a stage when the threat of intracranial haemorrhage has receded, the urge to obtain an urgent CT scan should be resisted. The unconscious or ventilated patient may develop atelectasis or lobar collapse. Without careful chest physiotherapy these developments lead to bronchopneumonia.

The multiply injured patient is at risk of developing the **Adult Respiratory Distress Syndrome**—commonly 2–4 days after injury. Many factors may contribute to this condition, including shock, overtransfusion with crystalloid fluids, sepsis, chest injury, and aspiration of vomit.

Fat embolus, complicating skeletal injuries, also develops after days or weeks, but characteristically between 24 and 48 hours after injury. The first manifestation of this syndrome may be a deteriorating conscious level or epileptic fits. The characteristic physical signs of fat embolus should be sought, and the arterial blood gases should be analysed. Oxygen therapy may be sufficient to improve the conscious level; but on occasions positive pressure ventilation will be required. This condition occurs most commonly in the young victims of multiple trauma, and the potential consequences for the brain injury are grave. Ideally, patients with this combination of problems should be observed in an Intensive Care Unit, so that prompt action is taken in the event of failing respiratory efficiency.

Ventilation must continue until the respiratory complications have resolved. This will be judged by serial chest X-rays and arterial blood-gas analysis, and by the nature and quantity of tracheal secretions.

Blood-volume depletion

Hypotension due either to blood loss or to impaired cardiac output leads to further impairment of cerebral perfusion. A deterioration in conscious level after head injury may be due to continuing blood loss from a variety of sources. Remember that the parameters for shock must be re-set in the patient with severe head injury (Chapter 3). Hypotension is rarely due to the head injury itself, unless there has been a very major scalp laceration.

> **Raised intracranial pressure may mask the signs of shock**.

It is easy to underestimate the extent of blood loss at the time of admission, and in the seriously injured patient it is important to repeat the haemoglobin and haematocrit measurements after volume replacement has been completed. Once haemodilution has taken place the haemoglobin may fall dramatically.

While a degree of haemodilution may be beneficial to cerebral perfusion by reducing viscosity this process, if continued, may lead to levels of circulating haemoglobin insufficient to maintain tissue oxygenation. Therefore, blood losses should be replaced with the aim of maintaining a haemoglobin level of at least 10g/100ml and a haematocrit of 30–35 per cent.

Obstruction of cerebral venous return

Obstruction of the venous outflow from the head causes elevation of the intracranial pressure and neurological deterioration. This can be caused by tilting the patient 'head-down' for counter-traction or for the insertion of central venous lines. The same effect can be caused by a tight cervical collar in the unconscious patient, and these should be removed as soon as the integrity of the cervical spine is established. This is especially important in the patient who has been paralysed for ventilation and in whom the neurological deterioration caused by the collar is not evident without an intracranial-pressure monitor.

Similar increases in intracranial pressure due to cerebral venous obstruction will result from attempts to intubate the unconscious patient who is capable of resisting. Unless the patient is so deeply unconscious that intubation can be carried out without any difficulty and without provoking gagging and coughing it is necessary to induce anaesthesia (see p. 144).

Epileptic fits

• Status epilepticus

Post-traumatic fits can complicate both severe head injuries and minor head injuries alike. Following the fit there is often a period of reduced consciousness, and if the patient is carefully observed it will become evident that the conscious level is improving. The occurrence of a fit is associated with a small increase in the incidence of intracranial haematoma; but there are always other indications that the patient is developing an intracranial mass. It is not to the advantage of a patient who has just had a fit to be promptly transferred by ambulance to a Neurosurgical Centre, on the assumption that the event heralds a developing intracranial haematoma. The main risk to the patient is that of respiratory embarrassment in the course of a further fit, and this is difficult to manage in a speeding ambulance.

In the event of a fit the main requirement is to guard the patient's airway. Most fits are self-limiting; but status epilepticus and frequent recurrent fits cause anoxic injury to the brain, and must be controlled. If it is clear that the clonic phase of the fit is slowing and the fit is going to cease spontaneously it is unnecessary to make any attempt to arrest it. The drugs used to treat status epilepticus are sedative and respiratory-depressant, and their effects complicate subsequent observation of conscious level.

Status epilepticus

If a fit persists for more than 2–3 minutes it should be arrested. The drugs in common use for this purpose are **diazepam** and **chlormethiazole**. Diazepam is the most convenient to use, and is administered by slow intravenous injection. It should be given in small aliquots, titrating the dose against the response. Chlormethiazole is administered by intravenous infusion. Both drugs are respiratory-depressants, and may cause serious respiratory depression or respiratory arrest even in the small doses used in the head-injured patient. They should only be used when facilities are available to ventilate the patient in the event of a respiratory arrest.

A single intravenous injection of diazepam may be sufficient to control status epilepticus. Treatment should continue with one of the anticonvulsant drugs listed in Box 4.3. Recurrent attacks of status epilepticus or frequent recurrent fits must be controlled by an intravenous infusion of either diazepam or chlormethiazole. Respiration must be closely monitored, and assisted ventilation may be required. The sedation caused by this treatment makes clinical monitoring of the patient's neurological condition difficult, and a CT scan should be performed in order to exclude an intracranial haematoma.

> **Sedative drugs may cause respiratory depression in the head-injured patient.**

After a single self-limiting fit the patient should be started on a regular anticonvulsant drug (Box 4.3). In the case of the unconscious patient or the patient with multiple injuries anticonvulsant drugs must be administered parenterally, and this limits the choice of drug to **phenytoin, sodium valproate**, and **phenobarbitone**. The first two drugs are the more commonly used, and in terms of their therapeutic value they are equally effective. Sodium valproate should not be used in women of child-bearing age. Phenytoin and sodium valproate are administered intravenously by slow injection (over 3–5 minutes). Because phenytoin may cause cardiac arrhythmias and hypotension, blood-pressure and ECG monitoring should be used when the drug is administered intravenously. Phenobarbitone should be given intramuscularly. In each case, a loading dose or a series of loading doses are given in order to establish therapeutic blood concentrations, followed by regular maintenance doses orally or parenterally. If the patient is expected to be able to take oral medication within the next 12 hours carbamazepine may be used instead of the drugs mentioned above. Anticonvulsant therapy in children is discussed in Chapter 8.

Box 4.2 Treatment of status epilepticus in adults

Diazepam	0–10 mg i.v. in 1 mg aliquots (titrate against effect)
	i.v. infusion 10–40 mg/hour
Chlormethiazole	0.8 per cent solution i.v. infusion 50–100 ml/hour until fits controlled

---

Box 4.3 Treatment of fits in adults

Phenytoin	250 mg i.v. (slow i.v. injection)
	250 mg i.v. t.d.s. for 24 hours
	100 mg i.v. t.d.s.
	300 mg oral/day when capable
Phenobarbitone	120 mg i.m.
	60 mg i.m. or oral t.d.s.
Sodium valproate	400–800 mg i.v. over 3–5 minutes
	200 mg i.v. or orally t.d.s.
Carbamazepine	200 mg b.d. increasing to 200 mg q.d.s.

Intracranial haematoma

- **Extradural haematoma**   Subdural haematoma
  Intracerebral haematoma

Intracranial haematoma is the only cause of neurological deterioration after head injury that requires operative neurosurgical intervention. The clinical features of an expanding intracranial mass are essentially the same whether it is a subdural, an extradural, or an intracerebral haematoma. The physiological effects of rising intracranial pressure are described in Chapter 1. The outcome of treatment is determined by the severity of the primary brain injury and the size and rapidity of onset of the haematoma.

Extradural haematoma

Extradural haemorrhage arises from meningeal blood vessels —commonly the middle meningeal vessels— and is the result of a skull injury. Approximately 90 per cent of adult patients with extradural haematoma have demonstrable skull fractures on X-ray. The recognition of a skull fracture, then, is most important in anticipating deterioration due to extradural haematoma. However, in children there is a lower incidence of radiologically recognized skull fracture in association with extradural haematoma (60–70 per cent).

The commonest site for extradural haematomas is in the temporal region, where the skull is thin and the middle meningeal vessels are vulnerable; but haematomas occur at other sites, usually determined by the site of the fracture. The haematoma caused by extradural haemorrhage strips the dura from the inner table of the skull as it increases in volume, and compresses the underlying brain. The effects of the haematoma are due to rising intracranial pressure and localized distortion of the brain.

Since this condition is so often associated with a relatively minor primary injury it is a particular tragedy if it is not recognized and treated.

Symptoms

The primary brain injury may have been minor, and, on

occasions, the patient may not have been unconscious at all. In either event, there is often a 'lucid interval' in which the patient may recover consciousness or remain conscious for a number of hours. This period is succeeded by increasing headache, vomiting, and deteriorating consciousness. Focal neurological deficits such as limb weakness or dysphasia may be recognized by the patient or by those in attendance. On some occasions, severe persistent headache alone, without altered consciousness or focal deficit, may be the mode of presentation. Extradural haemorrhage does, of course, also occur in the context of the severe primary injury, in which case it causes further deterioration in the already unconscious patient.

Examination
Associated with the skull fracture there may be a scalp injury. Subgaleal bleeding may give rise to a 'boggy' scalp haematoma. Consciousness may be depressed on the Glasgow Coma Scale; but some patients present with headache and focal neurological signs alone. There may be a contralateral limb weakness or evidence of dysphasia. As the haematoma develops the rising intracranial pressure is accompanied by bradycardia and hypertension, and increasing irregularity of respiration. Eventually the volume of the haematoma causes herniation of the ipsilateral temporal lobe through the tentorial hiatus, where it impinges on the oculomotor (third cranial) nerve. At this critical stage the ipsilateral pupil becomes dilated, and then ceases to react to light (Fig. 4.1).

Any further increase in the volume of the haematoma will result in dilatation of the contralateral pupil, and, unless treatment is instituted immediately, there is little likelihood of recovery.

Extradural haematomas in the posterior fossa cause rapid deterioration in consciousness and respiratory depression. Tachycardia and hypotension may be seen, in contrast to the findings in supratentorial haematomas.

Diagnosis
Neurological deterioration in the presence of a skull fracture is suggestive of an extradural haematoma. The site of the

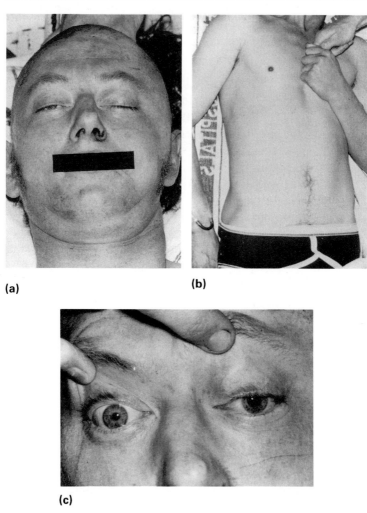

(a)

(b)

(c)

Fig. 4.1 • (a) Right-sided facial weakness in a patient with a left extradural haematoma. (b) Right-limb weakness in a patient with a left extradural haematoma. The right-hand limbs fail to move in response to a painful stimulus. (c) Dilated left pupil in a patient with a left extradural haematoma.

Box 4.4 **Clinical features of intracranial haematoma**

• Headache, vomiting
• Deteriorating conscious level
• Progressive hemiparesis (contralateral)
• Bradycardia, hypertension
• Dilating pupil (ipsilateral)
• Irregular respiration

scalp injury and the lateralization of the neurological signs indicate whether the lesion is on the left or the right. The haematoma is usually related to the site of the fracture. An extradural haematoma has a characteristic CT scan appearance (Fig. 4.2); but when scanning facilities are not available it may be necessary to proceed to surgery on the basis of the clinical signs and the skull X-ray.

Treatment
The definitive treatment of extradural haematoma requires a craniotomy, in order to remove the haematoma and control bleeding. It is desirable, and possible in most parts of the British Isles, that this should be done in a Neurosurgical Unit. Where distance or weather make transfer impossible the General Surgeon may have to be prepared to operate in the base hospital. If the patient's condition is deteriorating rapidly, or if the patient must be transferred to a distant hospital measures must be taken to prevent further deterioration in transit.

A temporary reduction in intracranial pressure can be achieved by intravenous administration of diuretic agents. Use either **mannitol** or **frusemide**. Mannitol is given as a rapid intravenous infusion, 0.5g being given per kg body weight. This amounts to 150–200 ml of a 20 per cent solution in an average adult, and it should be infused over 5 minutes. Frusemide is given as an intravenous bolus of 40 mg in an adult or 1 mg/kg body weight in a child. The ensuing diuresis will improve or at least hold the patient's condition, but only for 1–2 hours; and this treatment may

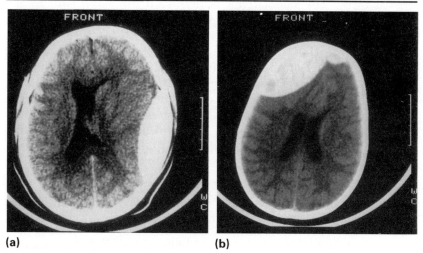

(a) **(b)**

Fig. 4.2 • (a) CT scan of a frontal extradural haematoma; (b) CT scan of a frontoparietal extradural haematoma.

have to be repeated if there is further deterioration before definitive investigations or treatment have been completed. During this time arrangements must be made as rapidly as possible to ensure that surgical treatment follows. Diuretics should **not** be given to hypovolaemic patients, since they will cause a further reduction in blood volume.

The deteriorating patient with an intracranial haematoma can ill afford any respiratory interruption, and should be anaesthetized, paralysed, and ventilated. Hyperventilation will also reduce intracranial pressure (see p. 14). This is an essential measure if the patient is to be transferred to a distant hospital.

Three units of blood should be cross-matched and available in the operating theatre.

A decision must then be made as to whether there is time to permit a CT scan. If not, the surgeon must decide on the site of the haematoma with the aid of the clinical signs and the skull X-ray. It should be remembered that a significant number of extradural haematomas are not found at the classical temporal site, but may be frontal or in the posterior fossa. The haematoma is found **on the same side as the dilated pupil** and on the **opposite** side to the hemiparesis. It is usually located **at the site of the skull fracture**.

An extradural haematoma is a solid clot covering a large area of the surface of the dura, and **cannot be treated through a burr-hole**. The ideal surgical procedure is a craniotomy: but, where the surgeon's experience does not permit this, a burr-hole can be extended to form a craniectomy by removing bone (see Chapter 9). This will be sufficient to save the patient's life; but the resulting skull defect will make further surgery necessary at a later date.

Box 4.5 Management of deteriorating patient with suspected intracranial haematoma

- Ensure that basic resuscitation is complete
- 20% mannitol i.v. bolus 0.5g/kg body weight
- Anaesthetize and ventilate
- Maintain paralysis and sedation
- Transfer if necessary
- Cross-match blood 3 units
- CT scan (if time permits)
- Craniotomy (craniectomy if craniotomy impossible)

The problems for the occasional surgeon operating outside a Neurosurgical Unit are that, firstly, the site of the lesion may be misjudged; and, secondly, the lesion may not prove to be the expected extradural haematoma, but an acute subdural or intracerebral haematoma. Furthermore, the main surgical challenge is not the removal of the clot, but the arrest of the subsequent bleeding, which can be extremely difficult for the uninitiated surgeon.

Operative surgical technique is discussed in Chapter 9.

Subdural haematoma

Subdural haematoma may be **acute** or **subacute**. The **acute subdural haematoma** is usually associated with a severe primary brain injury, causing further deterioration in the patient's already impaired conscious level and vital signs. The outcome will be determined substantially by the severity of the primary injury.

The **subacute subdural haematoma** develops over a period of days, and is due to haemorrhage from a bridging vein between the brain and the dura, often after relatively trivial trauma. In many instances this phenomenon is made possible by a degree of pre-existing cerebral atrophy. Thus it is commonly seen in alcoholics and the elderly. In the case of the former, alcoholic liver disease contributes the additional factor of impaired blood coagulation.

The clinical course of events is similar to that described for extradural haemorrhage, particularly in the case of the subacute haematoma which may present after a lucid interval. Similar focal neurological signs are seen, associated with bradycardia and hypertension. The finding of a skull fracture is less frequently associated with subdural haematoma.

Diagnosis

The clinical diagnosis of a subdural haematoma (as distinct from an extradural or intracerebral haematoma) cannot be made with any confidence. Its clinical localization is made according to the focal neurological signs (hemiparesis, dilated pupil); but it is impossible to predict on clinical grounds whether the lesion is frontal or parieto-occipital. Acute subdural haematoma has a characteristic CT scan appearance, and the scan allows the surgeon to determine the extent of the haematoma and to plan the surgical approach accordingly (see Fig. 4.3).

In the case of the alcoholic patient with a subacute haematoma it is wise to carry out clotting studies (prothrombin time, INR) and administer vitamin K 5 mg by slow intravenous injection preoperatively.

Treatment

While referral to a Neurosurgical Unit is being arranged the deteriorating patient can be stabilized by the use of intravenous mannitol 20 per cent and ventilation on the lines described for extradural haematoma.

Subdural haematoma is treated by craniotomy, and, since

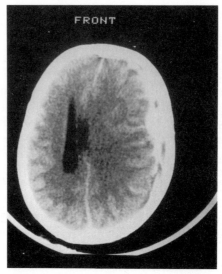

Fig. 4.3 • CT scan of an acute subdural haematoma with midline shift.

the site of origin of the haemorrhage cannot be determined preoperatively, a large craniotomy is required. If it is clear that the primary injury has been very severe and the patient presents with a very poor level of consciousness and un-reacting pupils, removal of the haematoma is unlikely to be followed by a useful recovery, and surgery is not indicated. Even in the case of the subacute haematoma results can be disappointing, because the pre-existing cerebral atrophy diminishes the brain's capacity for recovery.

Intracerebral haematoma

Traumatic intracerebral haematoma is, more strictly speak-ing, an area of haemorrhagic contusion caused by a closed-head injury, and often by the *contre-coup* mechanism. A common example is that of the patient who falls backwards and strikes the occiput. The frontal lobes are contused as they rebound off the frontal bone, and this may be followed by increasing swelling of the contused brain, leading to pro-gressive neurological deterioration.

The patient is usually ill with headache, focal neurological deficit, or altered consciousness from the time of the injury, and deteriorates over the course of days. The gradual deterioration may be missed if not carefully observed, until a critical point is reached, when the patient declines rapidly.

Diagnosis
As in the case of the subdural haematoma the nature and site of the lesion cannot be predicted clinically with confidence, and the diagnosis is made by CT scan.

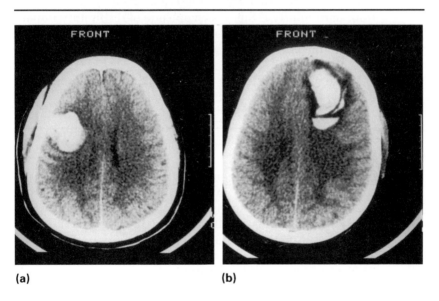

(a) **(b)**

Fig. 4.4 • (a) CT scan of a frontal intracerebral haematoma after occipital head injury; (b) CT scan of a left frontal intracerebral haematoma (the patient was struck by a golf ball).

These patients illustrate the dangers in operating on head-injured patients outside a Neurosurgical Unit without the aid of a scan. The fracture is remote from the haematoma, and the lesion is difficult to localize clinically. The inexperienced surgeon may be lead to operate at the wrong site, expecting to find an extradural haematoma at the site of the fracture.

Treatment

These patients require careful observation, preferably with intracranial-pressure monitoring. Since the lesion consists of contused brain, some of which may be viable, a conservative approach is followed unless the patient is clearly deteriorating. Swelling of the contused lobe may cause deterioration in the succeeding days, and this may take the form of a gradual deterioration in conscious level, hypertension and bradycardia, and increasing focal neurological deficit. On the other hand, there may be a rapid deterioration, particularly if there is an episode of respiratory impairment or an epileptic fit. It may then be necessary to carry out a craniotomy in order to evacuate the haematoma or to resect the injured lobe.

These patients should be observed in a Neurosurgical Unit, so that prompt treatment can be instituted.

Fluid balance

Overhydration and hyponatraemia may cause a deterioration in conscious level in the head-injured patient. Part of the early metabolic response to trauma is to retain water. The head-injured patient will often be breathing humidified oxygen, and insensible fluid-loss from respiration is largely abolished. **In the absence of other fluid-losses no more than 1500 cc of fluid will be required each day in adults.** While the patient is incapable of taking oral fluids daily fluid requirements should be supplied intravenously using a dextrose/saline combination.

After 3–4 days fluids may be given by nasogastric tube until the patient is capable of drinking. The head-injured patient is sensitive to water-overload, and over the course of 4 or 5 days of excessive fluids there may be a deterioration in conscious level. The diagnosis is confirmed by the finding of a low serum sodium. Hyponatraemia with a serum sodium of less than 130 mEq/l may also cause epileptic fits.

It is sufficient simply to stop all fluids until the excess water has been excreted, following which there may be a gradual but gratifying improvement in the patient's neurological condition. Do not give hypertonic saline. This simply exacerbates the problem of fluid overload.

Polyuria may occur for one of two reasons. The patient who is a known or latent diabetic may become hyperglycaemic in response to trauma. This is simply recognized if the urine is tested for sugar after admission. Or fractures of the base of the anterior cranial fossa may be complicated by injuries of the pituitary stalk, resulting in **diabetes insipidus**. If this is not recognized the patient may become seriously dehydrated and hypovolaemic. In this condition a low urine specific gravity and osmolality is associated with a high serum osmolality, a high haematocrit, and a high plasma sodium concentration. Careful fluid balance is important in the early stages of head-injury management.

Drugs

Sedative drugs should be avoided in the early stages after a head injury, while the patient's conscious level remains depressed. This means that opioid analgesics must be used with care (see p. 53). A deterioration in conscious level may be caused by opioid analgesics or by anticonvulsant agents. Establish whether any potentially sedative drugs have been given prior to deterioration.

> **Sedative drugs and opioids cause impairment of consciousness and respiratory depression.**

A not infrequent culprit is diazepam, administered during an epileptic fit, or, sometimes, even after a fit. The patient then fails to regain the former level of consciousness, and the problem may be compounded by respiratory depression, which, in turn, causes further cerebral depression. Diazepam and related drugs should not be administered to head-injured patients. The only exception to this rule is in the event of status epilepticus, when intravenous diazepam is justified as long as facilities are immediately available to intubate and ventilate the patient. **Flumazenil** is a specific antidote to benzodiazepines, and may be used if a deterioration in consciousness or respiration is thought to be due to diazepam or related drugs.

Sedative drugs are sometimes given to the head-injured patient who has become restless and uncooperative, having been drowsy and withdrawn initially. This turn of events signals a deterioration, not an improvement, in conscious level, and should raise the question of a developing intracranial haematoma. In these circumstances, sedation is potentially disastrous.

One of the cardinal reasons for admission of the head-injured patient to hospital is to protect the patient from further injury that may otherwise result from avoidable or treatable factors. This is made possible by monitoring conscious level and vital signs. The present chapter has outlined the possible causes of neurological deterioration; and it should be evident that in many instances systemic factors are responsible. Since these complications may require early treatment, it is important that precipitate transfer to a specialist unit should not replace adequate resuscitation.

Further reading

Jennett, B. and Carlin, J. (1978). Preventable mortality and morbidity after head injury. *Injury*, **10**, 31–9.

Jennett, Bryan and Galbraith, Sam (1984). *Introduction to neurosurgery*, Heinemann Medical, London.

Jennett, Bryan and Teasdale, Graham (1981). *Management of head injuries*, F. A. Davis Co., Philadelphia.

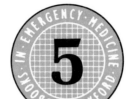

Chapter 5

Radiology

Key points in radiology

1 The main purpose of the skull X-ray in cases of trauma is to recognize a fracture and to establish whether or not it is a depressed fracture.

2 A linear fracture is seen as a hard black line, distinct from the normal marks, or as a widening of a suture line, particularly in children. A fracture, unlike vascular markings, may radiate in several directions from a central focus.

3 'Face-on', a depressed fracture is seen as a series of lines radiating from a central focus, or as a circular marking. Viewed tangentially, it is seen as a depression in the contour of the skull.

4 The extradural haematoma appears on a CT scan as a lens-shaped lesion that is convex inwardly.

5 The acute subdural haematoma appears on a CT scan as a layer of blood conforming to the surface of the cortex (i.e. concave inwardly).

6 The intracerebral haematoma appears on a CT scan as a patchy area of high density, with compression or shift of the ventricles, and clearly within the substance of the brain.

7 X-rays of the cervical spine should include lateral, antero-posterior, and, in the conscious patient, open-mouth views showing the odontoid process. The lateral view must include the C7–T1 junction, for which the patient's shoulders must be pulled down during X-ray.

8 The commonest sites for cervical-spine injuries are the C1/C2 region and the lower cervical spine (C5–C7), which should be examined on X-rays with particular attention.

9 A haematoma in the paraspinal tissues is seen on the lateral projection as an increase in the pre-spinal soft-tissue shadow (greater than 10 mm at the C1/C2 level, and 20 mm at the C5/C6 level in the adult).

The interpretation of skull X-rays often devolves to relatively junior doctors in the Accident and Emergency Department, often at hours when experienced colleagues are not always available. The finding of a skull fracture is important in its own right, in view of the possible complications of the skull injury. It is also important evidence that the patient has had a head injury when no history of trauma is available—for example, when a patient is admitted in an unconscious state of unknown aetiology.

Meningitis, subarachnoid haemorrhage, and epileptic fits may each be due to head trauma and, where no reliable history is available, skull X-rays are required in case the patient is presenting with one of these complications of head injury.

The head injury may be accompanied by injuries of the cervical spine, and a series of cervical-spine X-rays should be obtained in any conscious patient with neck pain and in all patients with altered consciousness.

Box 5.1   **Indications for skull X-ray**

- History of unconsciousness
- Scalp bruising, haematoma, laceration
- Neurological deficit
- Impaired conscious level
- CSF rhinorrhoea, otorrhoea
- Headache, vomiting
- Unconscious, ? head injury

Indications for skull X-rays

Skull X-rays are not indicated in all of the very large number of patients attending hospitals each year with head injuries. Undoubtedly, a very large number of normal skull X-rays are carried out every year, and of those that are found to have a skull fracture a small minority develop complications. The complications of the skull injury, however, are both lethal and either treatable or preventable, and the expense on radiology has to be viewed in this light. Various attempts have been made to rationalize the indications for skull X-rays; but, of course, guidelines are only guidelines, and the attending doctor must judge whether the skull is likely to have been injured according to the nature and severity of the injury.

The normal skull X-ray

- **The antero-posterior skull X-ray   The lateral skull X-ray   The Townes view**

In order to recognize abnormalities on the skull X-ray it is necessary to be familiar with the normal radiological anatomy of the skull in each of the conventional projections. When skull X-rays are requested, three views should be provided—an antero-posterior, a lateral, and a Townes projection. On each of these there are certain features which are constant in position, and others that are normal findings, but of variable position and appearance.

Where a depressed fracture is suspected, a tangential view of the area should be taken, so that the suspect area is placed on the 'sky-line' of the skull.

The normal markings seen on the skull vault are the **diploic veins** of the skull, the **meningeal vessels**, and the **suture lines**. The diploic veins are inconstant in position, and are seen as broad, soft markings. The **middle meningeal vessels** are constant in position, and more clearly demarcated. They can usually be seen to divide into anterior and posterior branches. Suture lines are characteristically 'saw-toothed' in appearance, and constant in position.

The antero-posterior skull X-ray

The normal AP skull X-ray (Fig. 5.1) shows the orbital margins, the frontal and ethmoid sinuses, the sagittal suture, and the lambdoid sutures, as well as the diploic veins.

The pineal gland may be seen as a calcified structure just above the eyebrows in the midline.

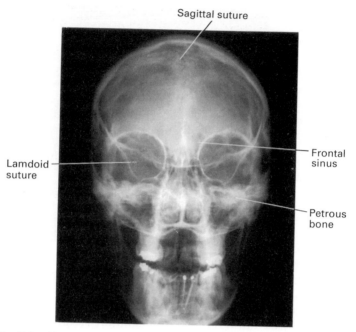

Sagittal suture

Lamdoid
suture

Frontal
sinus

Petrous
bone

Fig. 5.1 • Normal skull X-ray: antero-posterior view.

The lateral skull X-ray

The normal lateral skull X-ray (Fig. 5.2) shows the frontal sinuses and the sphenoid sinus. The other 'fixed' features are the coronal suture and the middle meningeal artery, which divides into an anterior and a posterior branch. The other normal features are the diploic veins of the skull, which are randomly distributed, and are seen as soft shadows. The pineal gland is often calcified, and is seen just above the pinna of the ear. If it is clearly visible on this view it may also be identifiable on the AP or Townes views, where it is more difficult to recognize.

The Townes view

This fronto-occipital projection shows the occipital bone.

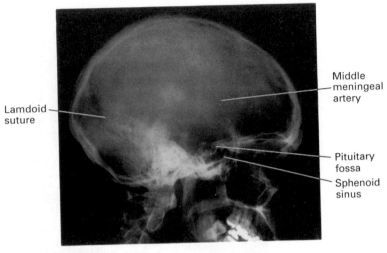

Fig. 5.2 • Normal skull X-ray: lateral view.

Note the normal features, which include the lambdoid sutures and the foramen magnum. The pineal gland may be visible as a midline calcified structure (Fig. 5.3).

The abnormal skull X-ray (skull fractures)

The main purpose of the skull X-ray in cases of trauma is to recognize a fracture and to establish whether it is a depressed fracture. Of occasional value is the demonstration of a shift of midline structures by showing a lateral displacement of a calcified pineal gland.

A linear fracture is seen as a hard black line, distinct from the normal markings (Fig. 5.4). Alternatively, there may be widening of a suture line, particularly in children. A fracture, unlike vascular markings, may radiate in several directions from a central focus. Skull fractures remain radiologically evident for many years after injury, and it can be impossible to determine whether a fracture is recent or old unless previous X-rays are available for comparison.

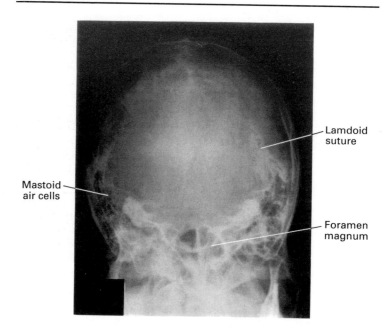

Fig. 5.3 • Normal skull X-ray: Townes view.

'Face-on', a depressed fracture is seen as a series of lines radiating from a central focus, or as a circular marking. Viewed tangentially, it is seen as a depression in the contour of the skull. The inner table of the skull may be depressed to a greater extent than the outer, and spicules of bone can be seen angled inwards (Fig. 5.5).

Fractures of the skull-base are often very difficult to detect on the standard projections above, and are recognized by indirect evidence. Since these fractures often involve the air sinuses they may result in blood or CSF occupying the sinuses. Typically, the sphenoid sinus is seen to contain fluid, which appears as an air–fluid level. Since the lateral skull view is taken with the patient lying horizontally and brow-up, the fluid level is best recognized by viewing the X-ray in this position (Fig. 5.6).

In basal skull fractures involving the sinuses and other

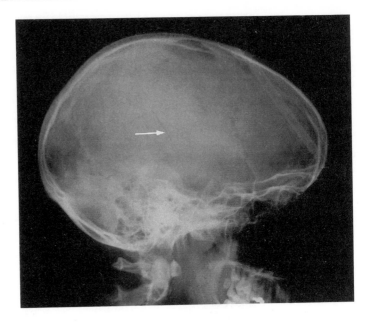

Fig. 5.4 • Abnormal skull X-ray: linear fracture.

compound injuries, penetration of the dura allows escape of CSF and entry of air into the cranial cavity. This is seen as black 'bubbles' within the skull. In the case of an anterior fossa fracture with CSF rhinorrhoea a large quantity of air may occupy the anterior fossa as an aerocele (Fig. 5.7).

The CT scan

- **Extradural haematoma   Subdural haematoma Intracerebral haematoma/contusion   Diffuse brain injury**

The indications for a CT scan are described in Chapter 3. In many instances it is necessary to transport the patient to another hospital if a scan is required. It is vital to ensure that

(a)

Depressed fracture

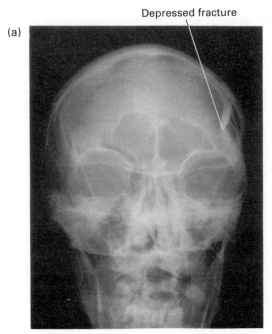

(b)

Depressed fracture

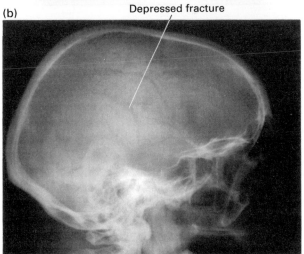

Fig. 5.5 • Abnormal skull X-ray: depressed fracture. (a) Frontal view; (b) lateral view.

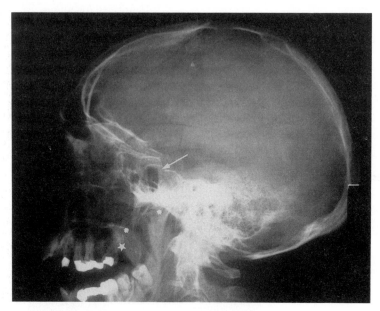

Fig. 5.6 • Abnormal skull X-ray: air–fluid level in a sinus.

the patient has been resuscitated adequately before being moved. Close observation and resuscitation facilities remain necessary during the scan. It is impossible to scan a moving patient, and in the case of the very restless patient a decision has to be taken as to whether to carry out the scan under general anaesthetic or to adopt a close watching policy and proceed to the scan if the patient's conscious level deteriorates or any focal neurological signs develop. The latter course is more safely conducted in a Neurosurgical Unit. Sedation with Diazepam or other similar agents should not be used, because of the serious danger of inducing respiratory depression.

> **Do not sedate the restless patient for a CT scan.**

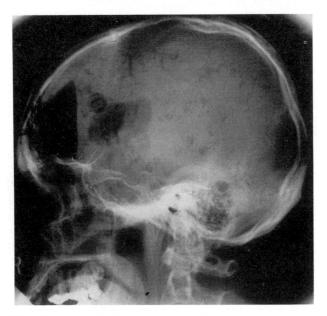

Fig. 5.7 • Abnormal skull X-ray: an aerocele.

Figs. 4.2, 4.3, and 4.4 show examples of CT abnormalities (pp. 71, 74, 75, respectively).

Extradural haematoma

Note that the extradural haematoma appears on a CT scan as a lens-shaped lesion that is convex inwardly. The associated skull fracture may be evident on the scan. The degree of ventricular shift gives an indication of the extent of the mass effect of the haematoma.

Subdural haematoma

The acute subdural haematoma appears on a CT scan as a layer of blood conforming to the surface of the cortex (i.e. concave inwardly).

Intracerebral haematoma/contusion

The intracerebral haematoma following trauma is usually a haemorrhagic contusion in which brain and blood are mixed to varying degrees. It is rarely a discrete clot. It appears on a CT scan as a patchy area of high density, with compression or shift of the ventricles, and is clearly within the substance of the brain.

Diffuse brain injury

Diffuse brain injury without extracerebral or intracerebral haematoma may present with CT evidence of brain swelling alone. The ventricles appear smaller than would be expected, taking into consideration the age of the patient. The basal cisterns may be effaced or absent. Small areas of haemorrhage may be seen scattered throughout the brain, but particularly in the corpus callosum. Severe diffuse brain injury may occur without any unequivocal abnormality on the CT scan.

X-rays of the cervical spine

- **Interpretation   CT scan of the cervical spine**
  Radiological assessment of stability

The initial X-rays of the cervical spine must be obtained without moving the patient from the resuscitation trolley. Routine examination of the cervical spine should include a lateral view, an antero-posterior view, and, in the conscious patient, an open-mouth view, to show the odontoid process. The lateral view must include the junction of C7 and T1. To achieve this the patient's shoulders must be pulled down by applying traction to the arms while the X-ray is taken. If this fails to demonstrate the lower cervical spine a 'swimmer's view' should be obtained by raising one of the arms above the head while the other is held downwards and behind the patient's back. These X-rays will show deformity of the spine, fractures of the vertebral bodies, and loss of normal alignment, and are sufficient for the early stages of management. Further views may be required later if the patient complains of symptoms such as neck pain or paraesthesia in the limbs.

The commonest sites for cervical-spine injuries are the C1/C2 region and the lower cervical spine (C5–C7). Particular attention should be paid to those areas when the X-rays are examined.

Interpretation

The X-rays must be examined, firstly, for evidence of a spinal injury, and, secondly, for evidence of instability. Examine each of the vertebral bodies in turn in the AP and lateral projections, noting obvious fractures or any alteration of the normal oblong outline (Fig. 5.8). Small triangular fragments may be avulsed from the anterior borders of the vertebral body in potentially unstable injuries without loss of alignment. In the lateral projection examine the spinous processes for fractures. Examine the open-mouth view for evidence of fractures of the odontoid process (Fig. 5.9).

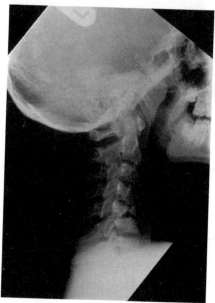

Fig. 5.8 • Abnormal cervical-spine X-ray: a vertebral fracture.

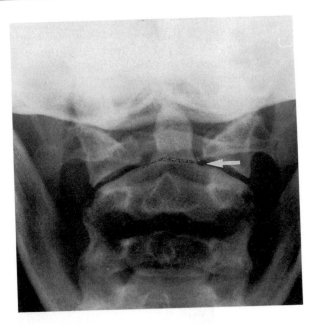

Fig. 5.9 • Open-mouth X-ray: a fracture of the odontoid process.

Inspect the lateral and AP views for loss of alignment. In the lateral projection the anterior and posterior surfaces of the vertebrae form a smooth anteriorly curving line. An abrupt loss of continuity in these lines indicates a subluxation or dislocation of the spine at this level (Fig. 5.10).

The disc spaces should also be examined. Widening of the disc space either anteriorly or posteriorly indicates disruption of the anterior or posterior longitudinal ligaments, and potential instability. Narrowing of the disc space may occur if there has been traumatic rupture of the disc.

At the level of the injury there may be a haematoma in the paraspinal tissues. This is seen on the lateral projection as an increase in the pre-spinal soft-tissue shadow. At the C1/C2 level, the soft-tissue shadow should not exceed 10 mm in the adult, and at the C5/C6 level it should be less than 20 mm. An increase in the soft-tissue shadow may be seen in the

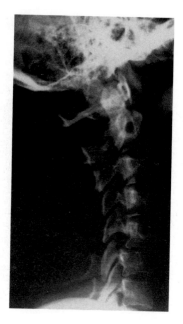

Fig. 5.10 • Abnormal cervical-spine X-ray: a loss of alignment in the spine.

absence of any obvious fracture or loss of alignment (Fig. 5.11).

If, after the standard views, there remains suspicion of a spinal injury further X-rays may be indicated. Oblique 45° views show the pedicles and facet joints, which are less readily defined on the AP and lateral projections. Conventional tomography and views in flexion and extension may be indicated.

CT scan of the cervical spine

Computed tomography has made an important contribution to the evaluation of the injured cervical spine. A number of fractures which cannot be demonstrated by conventional radiography are shown by CT scanning. Furthermore, CT is capable of demonstrating in detail the configuration of the fracture and its potential instability (Fig. 5.12).

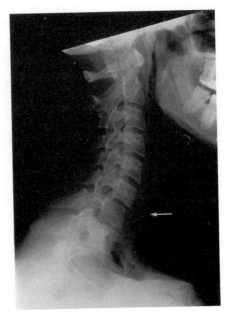

Fig. 5.11 • Abnormal cervical-spine X-ray: increased pre-spinal soft-tissue shadow.

Radiological assessment of stability

The stability of a cervical-spine injury depends on the site and configuration of fractures, the presence of ligamentous injuries, and the mechanism of the injury. Certain fractures must always be regarded as unstable. Fractures of the odontoid process belong to this category. Burst fractures of the vertebral bodies and fractures involving the facet joints or lateral masses of other vertebrae should be assumed to be unstable. Evidence of disruption of the anterior or posterior spinal ligaments or the interspinous ligaments with or without loss of alignment indicate potential instability. Ultimately, the stability of a particular fracture may have to be tested by carefully controlled flexion and extension views; but these should not be taken in the Accident and Emergency Depart-

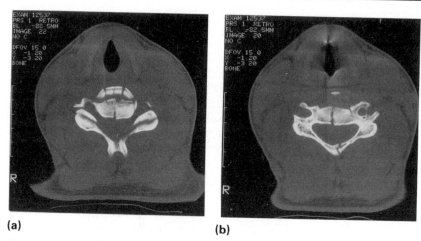

(a)   **(b)**

Fig. 5.12 • CT scan of a cervical-spine fracture. (a) Comminuted fracture of vertebral body; (b) fracture of vertebral body and lamina.

ment. The patient should be admitted under the care of a Neurosurgeon or Orthopaedic Surgeon, and flexion/extension views should be taken only after consultation with an experienced Radiologist.

Further reading

Anon. (1984). Guidelines for initial management after head injury in adults: suggestions from a group of neurosurgeons. *British Medical Journal*, **288**, 983–5.

Anon. (1987). Skull X-ray examinations after head trauma: recommendations by a multidisciplinary panel and validation study. *New England Journal of Medicine*, **316**, 84–91.

du Boulay, G. H. (ed.) (1977). *Computerised axial tomography in clinical practice*.

Meyer, P. R. (1989). *Surgery of spine trauma*, Chapter X. Churchill Livingstone Inc., New York.

Tyson, George W. (1987). *Head injury management for providers of emergency care*, pp. 121–68. Williams & Wilkins, Baltimore.

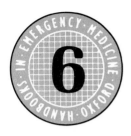

Chapter 6

Scalp and skull injuries

Key points in scalp and skull injuries

1 Bruising of the mastoid processes behind the ears is evidence of a fracture of the petrous bone, which in turn indicates the patient may be at risk of meningitis from a fracture communicating with the middle-ear cavity.

2 Extracranial haematomas are recognized as characteristically 'boggy' swellings in the scalp overlying the fracture.

3 Unless a careful clinical examination of the scalp (which is also important for medico-legal reasons) is carried out, serious penetrating injuries may easily be missed if the wound is small. Failure to recognize the possibility that a small scalp injury may be deeply penetrating may expose the patient to the risk of meningitis or cerebral abscess.

4 The scalp of a child with a subgaleal haematoma is tense and fluctuant, and the child may be distressed, restless, and febrile. The haematoma can be aspirated with a syringe and a large-bore needle, but only in an operating theatre with full aseptic precautions—not as an outpatient procedure.

5 Where scalp lacerations involve skin-loss or are cosmetically important wounds should be closed by a plastic surgeon, as wound closure without tension can become very difficult. Heavy blood-loss is to be expected.

6 'Scalping' injuries involve serious blood-loss, and there is a danger the skin flap may become ischaemic.

7 Skull-base fractures in the anterior fossa are recognized clinically by the presence of periorbital haematomas or subconjunctival haemorrhages, and by evidence of CSF rhinorrhoea. They may be complicated by meningitis: therefore the patient should be treated with prophylactic antibiotics for one week from the time of injury or the cessation of CSF rhinorrhoea or otorrhoea.

8 Patients with scalp lacerations and underlying fractures should also be given prophylactic antibiotics.

9 Patients presenting with headache, fever, and focal neurological signs some weeks or months after a penetrating head injury should excite a suspicion of a subdural empyema. Meningism may be present, but the presence of focal signs should deter lumbar puncture until empyema has been excluded—the raised ICP of empyema could render lumbar puncture lethal. Patients should be referred to a neurosurgeon if this diagnosis is suspected.

Scalp injuries

• **Significance of scalp injuries   Scalp lacerations**

Significance of scalp injuries

The scalp injury both draws attention to the fact that the patient has had a head injury and may itself be of serious significance. Failure to recognize that the patient has had a head injury may mean that, in the event of deterioration, the possibility of intracranial haemorrhage is not considered.

The unconscious patient presenting in the Accident and Emergency Department may have had a head injury, and this is sometimes not clear from the history. A careful search of the scalp is an essential part of the examination in order to identify the signs of trauma. These may be relatively slight and obscured by hair. Gently palpate the whole scalp in order to recognize scalp haematomas, and part the hair to look for lacerations or contusions. Always look behind the ears for bruising of the mastoid processes, which is evidence of a fracture of the petrous bone; and this in turn indicates that the patient may be at risk of meningitis from a fracture communicating with the middle-ear cavity.

Skull fractures are associated with both extracranial and intracranial haemorrhage. Extracranial haematomas are recognized as characteristically **'boggy' swellings** in the scalp overlying the fracture. This may be easier for the novice to recognize than the radiological appearance of the fracture.

> **Scalp injuries draw attention to possible skull injuries.**

The scalp injury may be of some medico-legal significance, and it is important to record both the number of injuries and their appearance. Unless a careful clinical examination of the scalp is carried out serious penetrating injuries may easily be missed if the external wound is small. The patient whose X-ray is shown in Fig. 6.1 was not recognized to have a penetrating head injury until his skull was X-rayed.

Failure to recognize the possibility that a small scalp in-

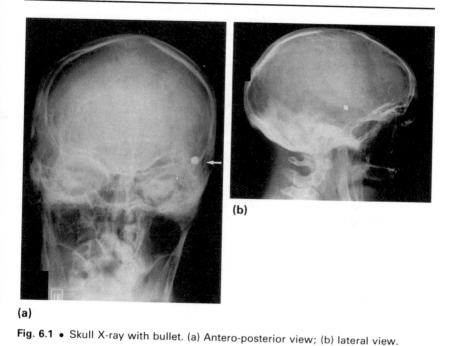

(b)

(a)

Fig. 6.1 • Skull X-ray with bullet. (a) Antero-posterior view; (b) lateral view.

jury may be deeply penetrating may expose the patient to the risk of meningitis or cerebral abscess.

In children, a scalp injury may be complicated by bleeding in the subgaleal layer of the scalp. The scalp of the patient with a **subgaleal haematoma** is tense and fluctuant. The condition can be very painful, and the child may be distressed, restless, and febrile. If this condition causes severe symptoms the haematoma should be aspirated with a syringe and a large-bore needle; but great caution should be exercised, since infection of the subgaleal haematoma is a serious complication. Aspiration should be carried out in an operating theatre with full aseptic precautions, and not as an outpatient procedure.

The younger the child the greater the proportion of the total blood volume that may be thus sequestrated in the scalp; and an infant with a large scalp haematoma may have lost a significant proportion of the circulating blood volume.

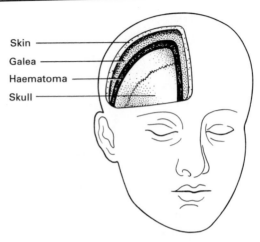

Skin
Galea
Haematoma
Skull

Fig. 6.2 • Diagram of scalp layers and subgaleal haematoma.

Scalp lacerations

The majority of scalp lacerations are simple linear lacerations requiring wound closure under local anaesthetic. More extensive lacerations are more appropriately dealt with under general anaesthesia. Where there are cosmetic considerations or where there is actual skin-loss this is best handled by a plastic surgeon, as even a relatively small loss of skin can make wound closure without tension extremely difficult.

The scalp is a very vascular structure, and the blood-loss from an extensive laceration can be considerable. The patient may be capable of compensating by vasoconstriction, only to reveal the extent of the blood-loss at the induction of anaesthesia, when the blood-pressure may drop alarmingly.

The scalp laceration affords an opportunity for the doctor to inspect the skull directly for fractures, and a careful inspection of the wound and palpation with a sterile gloved finger should always be performed to detect any underlying skull injury.

Management of scalp lacerations

For the majority of simple linear scalp lacerations it is sufficient to clean and suture the wound under local anaesthetic:

1 per cent **lignocaine** should be used combined with **adrenaline** 1/200 000.

During inspection and suturing of the wound blood-loss can be controlled by the pressure of an assistant's fingertips along the wound margins (Fig. 6.3). Bleeding will cease after the wound is sutured. It is inefficient and unnecessary to attempt to ligate individual bleeding-points.

As with wounds elsewhere, devitalized tissue should be exercised. If this is likely to leave a scalp defect that cannot be closed without tension it is quite acceptable to clean and dress the wound and seek Plastic Surgery advice. Where there is loss of skin it is necessary to be prepared to rotate a scalp flap and cover the donor area with a split skin-graft. This will require a general anaesthetic and a surgeon with Plastic Surgery experience. It is even more important to be sure of sound scalp-healing if there is an underlying fracture.

When it is anticipated that the wound may be difficult to close without tension it is wise to consider suturing the wound under general anaesthetic, since infiltration with local anaesthetic can further restrict the mobility of the skin edges.

Before suturing the wound the scalp should be shaved around the margins of the lacerations so that it can be adequately cleaned and the true extent of the injury can be seen.

Most scalp wounds can be closed with a single layer of interrupted non-absorbable sutures of 2/0 or 3/0 gauge. Sutures are usually removed after 5 days.

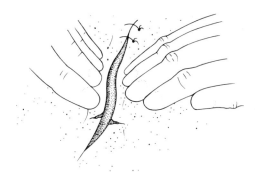

Fig. 6.3 • Finger pressure controlling scalp bleeding.

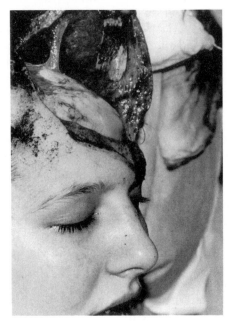

Fig. 6.4 • A scalping injury.

'Scalping' injuries are a rare but serious variety of scalp wound (Fig. 6.4). Where a large part of the scalp is avulsed there may be serious blood-loss, and there is a danger that the skin flap may be rendered ischaemic.

Skull injuries

- **Closed fractures Compound skull fractures Skull-base fractures: role of antibiotic prophylaxis Compound linear fractures of the skull vault Compound depressed fractures**

Skull fractures may be closed or compound, or linear or depressed, and may involve the skull vault or the skull base. The latter may involve the paranasal or mastoid air sinuses and the cranial nerves as they pass through the skull base. The fracture may require treatment in its own right, or may be significant because of its potential complications.

The presence of a skull fracture is among the important indications for admission to hospital after a head injury, and it is necessary to be able to recognize both the clinical and the radiological signs.

Like scalp injuries, skull fractures draw attention to the fact that the patient has had a head injury. A skull X-ray is a necessary investigation in the assessment of the unconscious patient when a reliable history is not available.

Closed fractures

The linear fracture does not require treatment in its own right. Both linear and depressed fractures, however, may be complicated by intracranial haemorrhage. Even in the conscious and orientated patient (i.e. those with Glasgow Coma Scores of 13–14) the presence of a skull fracture is associated with a risk of intracranial haematoma of 1 in 30, and these patients must be admitted to hospital for observation. The significance of the fracture is increased if the patient is not fully conscious. In these circumstances 1 in 4 patients will have some form of intracranial haematoma, and all such patients will require a CT scan.

> **Skull fractures may be complicated by extradural or other intracranial haematomas.**
>
> **Skull fracture together with altered consciousness indicates a 25 per cent chance of intracranial haematoma.**

The closed depressed fracture shares the properties of the linear fracture, but may also be disfiguring. This is usually when the fracture is situated outside the hair-line in the frontal region.

Depressed fractures elsewhere are generally covered by hair, and do not present a cosmetic problem. A disfiguring frontal depressed fracture requires to be elevated on

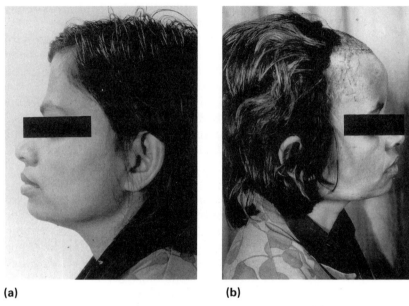

(a)   (b)

Fig. 6.5 • A depressed frontal fracture. (a) Before operation; (b) after operation.

cosmetic grounds; but a closed depressed fracture behind the hair-line can usually be left untreated.

Compound skull fractures

Skull fractures may be compound either when there is an overlying scalp wound, in which case the injury may penetrate the dura or brain, or if the fracture involves the air sinuses or the cribriform plate. In either case there is a risk of infective complications.

Skull-base fractures: role of antibiotic prophylaxis

Skull-base fractures in the anterior fossa are recognized clinically by the presence of periorbital haematomas or subconjunctival haemorrhages, and by evidence of CSF rhinorrhoea. The nature of the injury should also alert the doctor to the possibility of an anterior fossa fracture. Nasal and facial fractures are associated with damage to the skull base.

Fractures of the petrous bone may involve the middle-ear cavity and the mastoid air-cells. This may be clinically evident if there is bruising over the mastoid bone or blood, or CSF issuing from the external meatus.

Fractures of the petrous bone may also be accompanied by haemorrhage into the middle ear and disruption of the middle-ear apparatus, resulting in haemotympanum and deafness.

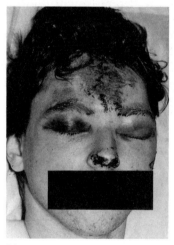

Fig. 6.6 • Periorbital haematomas.

The radiological detection of these fractures may be very difficult using standard views. Since these fractures involve the air sinuses, the cribriform plate, or the middle ear and mastoid air-cells, they may be complicated by persisting cerebrospinal fluid rhinorrhoea or otorrhoea, and by **meningitis** (see Chapter 10, pp. 168–70).

Skull-base fractures may be complicated by meningitis.

Antibiotic prophylaxis for skull-base fractures

When a skull-base fracture is diagnosed clinically or radiologically the patient should be treated with prophylactic antibiotics. The choice of antibiotics is determined by the expected pathogens and by the drug's ability to penetrate the blood–brain barrier. By far the most common organism involved in anterior fossa fractures is *Streptococcus pneumoniae*, which is a commensal organism in the nasopharynx. *S. pneumoniae* is usually sensitive to **benzyl penicillin**. **Erythromycin** is a suitable alternative in the case of penicillin allergy. It is necessary to consider whether the antibiotic is likely to penetrate the cerebrospinal fluid. Since sulphonamides do penetrate the cerebrospinal fluid effectively, an accepted combination for prophylaxis is benzyl penicillin or penicillin v with sulphadimidine 500 mg q.d.s. It is likely, however, that sulphadimidine will be withdrawn from the market in the near future; and a suitable substitute is co-trimoxazole.

A variety of commensal organisms are found in the middle ear, including Gram-negative and anaerobic species. Antibiotic prophylaxis should cover the possibility of infection by these organisms, and should provide a broad spectrum of antimicrobial activity. Metronidazole should be used in conjunction with either a cephalosporin or co-amoxiclav.

Box 6.1   Antibiotic prophylaxis in compound head injury

Anterior cranial fossa fracture		Benzyl penicillin
	or	penicillin v
	+	sulphadimidine
	or	co-trimoxazole
Petrous bone fracture		Metronidazole
	+	cephalosporin
	or	co-amoxiclav
Penetrating vault injury		Flucloxacillin
	or	Co-amoxiclav
	or	Cephalosporin

Although the use of prophylactic antibiotics is accepted practice in these circumstances there is little scientific evidence to indicate their effectiveness in preventing meningitis, or what is the ideal duration of treatment. The duration of treatment is, therefore, somewhat arbitrary; but it is commonly advised that antibiotic prophylaxis should continue for one week from the time of injury or for the same period after CSF rhinorrhoea or otorrhoea has ceased.

Compound linear fractures of the skull vault

It is important, when dealing with a scalp laceration, to establish whether there is an underlying fracture both by direct inspection and radiologically. Because of the potential complication of **meningitis** particular care should be exercised in ensuring that the wound is cleaned and soundly repaired. The patient should be given a course of prophylactic antibiotics. If the wound heals by first intention and without infection a one-week course is adequate. Since the pathogen is likely to be *Staphylococcus aureus* the choice of antibiotic should be flucloxacillin or co-amoxiclav or, in the case of penicillin allergy, a cephalosporin.

Compound depressed fractures

An innocent-looking laceration may be associated with a depressed fracture of the underlying skull. This should be recognized when the wound is explored or from the X-ray. Evidence of depression of the fracture may not be obvious unless a tangential view of the injured area of the skull is obtained (see Fig. 5.5, p. 87). Although, on direct inspection, the outer table of the skull may appear to be minimally depressed, the inner table may be much more depressed, with penetration of the underlying structures. These features may be more obvious on the skull X-ray or the CT scan (Fig. 6.7).

Penetrating brain injuries carry the additional risk of **cerebral abscess**, as depressed bone fragments may penetrate the meninges and the brain. Along with fragments of bone, hair, road dirt, and other debris may contaminate the

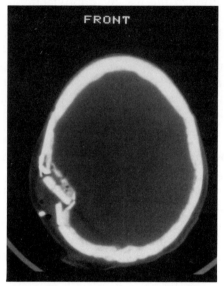

Fig. 6.7 • CT scan of a depressed parietal skull fracture.

wound. These injuries must be taken very seriously, since the complications are both easily avoided and potentially lethal.

> **All compound depressed fractures must be surgically explored.**

An inadequately treated compound head injury may also result in osteomyelitis of the skull and the relatively rare complication of **subdural empyema**. The patient usually presents with headache, fever, and focal neurological signs some weeks or even months after a penetrating head injury. Meningism may be present; but the history and the presence of focal signs should deter the doctor from carrying out a lumbar puncture until an empyema has been excluded. This condition causes raised intracranial pressure, which makes lumbar puncture potentially lethal. Subdural empyema can usually be recognized by CT scanning; but the CT appearances may be subtle, and a high index of clinical suspicion is important. If the diagnosis is suspected the patient should be referred to a neurosurgeon.

Some compound head injuries caused by high-velocity impacts or missile injuries may present a spectacular appearance, with exposure or extrusion of brain tissue through the fracture. These injuries are usually associated with more diffuse brain injuries, and it is important that the clinician is not distracted by the grotesque head wound to the detriment of the primary task of resuscitating the patient. The scalp wound should be dressed with cotton swabs and a bandage, and dealt with more definitively once the patient's condition has been stabilized. Urgent neurosurgical attention is therefore not primarily required at this stage, until the patient's resuscitation is complete.

Box 6.2 Complications of compound skull injury

- Meningitis
- Cerebral abscess
- Subdural empyema
- Aerocele

Compound depressed fractures must **always** be explored formally in the operating theatre. In the case of the simple laceration with a shallow depressed fracture it is sufficient to extend the wound and elevate the fracture so that the dura can be inspected for lacerations (see Operative surgery, Chapter 9). Care should be exercised in elevating fractures over one of the major venous sinuses; and it is unwise for the inexperienced surgeon to explore a depressed fracture in the midline of the head or over the occiput.

Penetrating brain injuries should be explored, and both debris and contaminated or devitalized tissues should be removed in order to prevent cerebral abscess.

Patients with penetrating head injuries should be treated with prophylactic antibiotics as described above. In the case of compound injuries of the skull vault the most likely contaminating organism is *Staphylococcus*, and the choice of antibiotic must be made with this in mind.

Complications of skull fracture

• CSF leakage   Cranial-nerve injuries

Cerebrospinal fluid leakage

Skull-base fractures may be complicated by leakage of cerebrospinal fluid into the paranasal air sinuses or the nose, in the case of anterior fossa fractures, and into the middle-ear cavity or the mastoid air-cells, in the case of petrous bone fractures. Fluid from the middle ear may pass from the Eustachian tube to the pharynx, presenting as rhinorrhoea.

When the discharge is bloodstained it may be difficult to be sure of the presence of cerebrospinal fluid, and it should then be assumed to be present. The patient should be admitted to hospital while the cerebrospinal fluid fistula persists. Antibiotics should be commenced as directed above. The patient should be advised not to blow the nose, since this increases the chance of introducing infection, and may, in addition, create an **aerocele** in the anterior fossa. This collection of air under pressure may cause severe headache, and is one cause of gradual or abrupt deterioration of conscious level in a patient with an anterior-fossa fracture.

In the majority of cases the fistula will close spontaneously. Antibiotics should be continued for a week after the discharge has ceased. When the discharge persists—and this is most commonly in cases of rhinorrhoea—surgical intervention should be considered in order to repair the dural defect. Opinions differ as to when this decision should be made; but most surgeons would intervene if the fistula persisted after ten days.

Cranial-nerve injuries

Fractures of the skull base may be complicated by cranial-nerve injuries. Cranial-nerve injuries also occur in the absence of fractures.

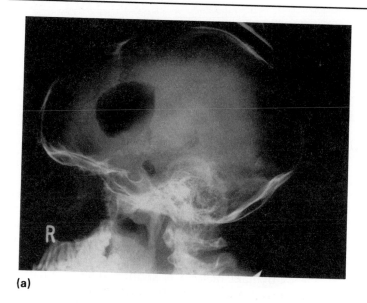

(a)

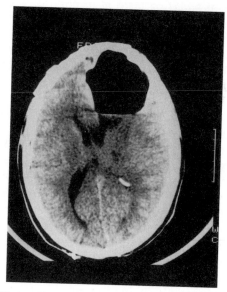

(b)

Fig. 6.8 • (a) X-ray of a frontal aerocele; (b) CT scan of a large frontal aerocele.

Box 6.3 **Complications of skull fracture**

- Intracranial haematoma
- Cerebrospinal fluid fistula
- Cranial-nerve injury
- Cosmetic deformity
- Aerocele

The olfactory nerves are injured in 5–10 per cent of closed head injuries. The impact causes shearing of the olfactory nerves as they pass through the cribriform plate; or the nerve may be injured in fractures of the anterior cranial fossa. The symptoms are usually of little concern to the patient in the immediate period after the injury; but on recovery the loss of the sense of smell can be distressing. Taste is impaired, and the enjoyment of food is spoiled. These impairments may also have implications in certain occupations where the sense of smell or taste is important. They are certainly regarded as a significant consequence of injury in subsequent litigation.

Optic-nerve injuries are mercifully uncommon. They tend to occur in severe frontal and facial injuries, such as are seen in road-traffic accidents when the front occupants of the car are thrown through the windscreen. The injury may involve the nerve itself or the optic chiasm. The visual fields must be assessed as soon as the patient is able to open the eyes. The light reflex may be absent or reduced; but the consensual reflex operates when the light is shone in the uninjured eye. The 'fixed pupil' in this case should not be confused with that resulting from a third (oculomotor) cranial-nerve lesion. The injured optic nerve is capable of recovering with time. Surgical intervention is not helpful.

Diplopia may be due either to injuries of the third, fourth, or sixth cranial nerves, or, more commonly, to bony injuries of the orbit. **The oculomotor (third) cranial nerve** may be injured directly by the impact. The pupil of the affected eye is dilated, and the light reflex is impaired. This is associated with a palsy of the extraocular muscles served by the third nerve, and occasionally with a ptosis. The extraocular palsy is most evident as a weakness of the medial rectus muscle. The patient complains of diplopia on looking to the side of the injured nerve. A dilated pupil also occurs in direct trauma to the eye, in which case there is usually no associated extraocular palsy, and there is evidence of direct trauma to the orbit in the form of bruising or abrasions on the orbital margins, conjunctival injuries, and intraocular blood. The patient with a direct eye injury or an isolated third-nerve injury will be conscious and otherwise relatively well. The patient who develops a third-nerve palsy as a result of an expanding intracranial mass, on the other hand, is not conscious, and has other signs associated with a severe head injury. The two situations should be readily distinguished.

Injuries of the **fourth (trochlear) nerve** and the **sixth (abducent) nerve** occur in 1–9 per cent of all head injuries. The former causes weakness of the superior oblique muscle and diplopia on downward gaze. The latter affects the lateral rectus muscle, and causes diplopia on gaze to the opposite side. Fortunately, injuries of the third, fourth, and sixth cranial nerves tend to resolve spontaneously. Diplopia is treated in the first instance by providing an eye-patch. If there is persisting diplopia this can be corrected by the provision of prism lenses.

The fifth (trigeminal) nerve is usually injured in fractures of the facial skeleton, resulting in numbness over the cheek.

The facial nerve is injured extracranially in direct blows to the pre-auricular area, and intracranially in fractures of the petrous bone. The facial palsy may be delayed, in which case it is presumed that the progressive facial palsy is attributable to swelling of the nerve within its canal. The extent of the palsy may be limited if the patient is given a short course of corticosteroids. **Prednisolone** 80 mg/day should be prescribed as early as possible after the facial weakness becomes apparent, and continued for 4 to 5 days. The drug should be stopped if there is no response at that stage, or phrased out gradually over a longer period if recovery is apparent. This injury is often associated with bruising of the mastoid, and there may be an accompanying injury of the middle ear and CSF otorrhoea.

Middle-ear injuries may result in deafness and bleeding from the external meatus. Inspection with the otoscope will show whether there is a laceration of the external meatus and whether there is a haemotympanum. Again, there is usually no immediate treatment required. A haemotympanum will resolve spontaneously; but persisting deafness may be due to injury of the **acoustic nerve** or the ossicles, and the patient should be referred for the opinion of an ENT surgeon.

Symptoms related to middle-ear and acoustic-nerve injuries are common after head injury, and frequently bring patients back to the Accident Department for advice.

Injuries of the lower cranial nerves occur rarely, and are due to fracture of the occipital bone in the region of the jugular and hypoglossal foramina.

Further reading

Braakman, R. (1972). Depressed skull fracture: data, treatment and follow-up in 225 consecutive cases. *Journal of Neurology, Neurosurgery, and Psychiatry*, **35**, 396–402.

Leech, P. (1974). Cerebrospinal fluid leakage, dural fistulae and meningitis after basal skull fracture. *Injury*, **6**, 141–9.

Tyson, G. W. (1987). *Head injury management for providers of emergency care*, pp. 120–35. Williams & Wilkins, Baltimore.

Vinken, P. J. and Bruyn, G. W. (eds) (1969). *Handbook of clinical neurology*, vol. 24 (cranial nerve injuries).

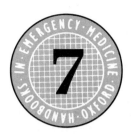

Chapter 7

Cervical-spine
injuries

Key points in cervical-spine injuries

1 All unconscious patients must be assumed to have injuries of the cervical spine.

2 If an accident victim is suspected of having a cervical-spine injury every effort must be made to immobilize the neck before the patient is moved at the scene of the accident, using a hard collar that can be applied in two pieces and makes contact with chin and occiput superiorly and sternum and shoulders inferiorly.

3 Three persons are needed to lift the patient without manipulation of the spine, one of them controlling the head and neck.

4 Once the patient has been placed on the ambulance trolley as little subsequent movement as possible should be allowed until the integrity of the cervical spine has been established.

5 Priapism is an ominous sign associated with complete spinal-cord injury—a possibility which should also be considered if the unconscious patient makes no response to a painful stimulus. Hypotension and bradycardia may also be seen.

6 In cases of partial spinal-cord and unstable spinal injury muscle-power and sensation must be tested hourly for the first 24 hours.

7 If a cervical-spine injury is thought to be unstable skull traction must be applied, as it should where there is loss of alignment due to fracture or dislocation, under the supervision of an experienced Orthopaedic Surgeon or Neurosurgeon.

8 Urgent surgery should be reserved for patients who show progressive deterioration due to spinal-cord compression by prolapsed intervertebral-disc material or haematoma, and for unstable ligamentous injuries in the absence of a spinal-cord lesion, which tend to remain unstable unless some form of bony fusion is undertaken.

In the victims of trauma, the head and neck should be considered as a single unit. The forces that are responsible for head injuries also cause injuries of the cervical spine, and the two conditions are commonly associated. In one autopsy series of 312 fatal road-traffic accidents, 10 per cent of cases had combined head and cervical-spine injuries.

Conscious patients are able to report symptoms associated with cervical-spine trauma but, in the light of the statistics presented above, all unconscious patients must be assumed to have injuries of the cervical spine. This governs the management of the patient from the time of the accident.

Immediate immobilization of the cervical spine

If an accident victim is suspected of having a cervical-spine injury every effort must be made to immobilize the neck before the patient is moved at the scene of the accident. This is best achieved using a hard collar that can be applied in two pieces and fixed by Velcro strapping. Soft collars are not adequate. Ideally, the collar should make contact with the chin and the occiput superiorly, and the sternum and shoulders inferiorly. If the patient is unconscious a tightly-applied cervical collar may exacerbate raised intracranial pressure by compressing the jugular veins. A variety of collar designs are available.

When the patient is moved the head and neck must be controlled. Three persons are necessary to lift the patient without manipulation of the spine. A fourth individual must remain responsible for controlling the head and neck (Fig. 7.1).

Once the patient has been placed on the ambulance trolley as little subsequent movement as possible should be allowed until the integrity of the cervical spine has been established. The patient can be placed on a spinal board or Scoop stretcher, and left on this surface during initial examination and resuscitation.

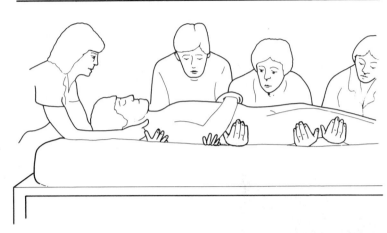

Fig. 7.1 • Drawing of a three-person lift, also showing a fourth person stabilizing the neck.

Clinical assessment of the spinal injury

• **History and examination**

Once the airway has been cleared and respiration and blood volume have been stabilized X-rays of the cervical spine must be obtained. Antero-posterior and lateral views are obtained without moving the patient from the resuscitation trolley. If these views are normal an unstable injury of the cervical spine is unlikely, but is not excluded altogether; and the neck must still be controlled when the patient is moved. Radiological assessment of the cervical spine is discussed in Chapter 5.

History and examination

If the patient is conscious ask about symptoms suggesting cervical-spine injury. Enquire about neck pain, paraesthesia, and limb weakness. Establish when the patient last emptied the bladder. If the patient is unconscious ask witnesses whether the patient was seen to move all four limbs after the accident. On inspection, note persistent rotation of the neck, indicating unilateral facet dislocation. Facial injuries suggest the possibility of a hyperextension injury of the neck. Observe spontaneous limb movements in the unconscious patient. Priapism is an ominous sign associated with complete spinal-cord injury. If the unconscious patient makes no response to a painful stimulus consider the possibility that there is a complete cervical spinal-cord injury. The patient with high cord injuries retaining only proximal upper limb power may be seen to lie with the upper limbs flexed.

If the patient is able to co-operate, carry out a detailed neurological examination as soon as initial resuscitation has been completed. Using a pin, test pain-sensation on both sides of the body, in an orderly pattern from the occiput to the perineum. In the case of a complete spinal-cord injury a sensory level is found, below which sensation is absent. In the incomplete spinal-cord injury sensory changes may be more subtle, and, in place of a sensory level below which all sensation is absent, there may be a level below which the quality of pain-sensation is altered—the pinprick being felt as a blunt touch. On rare occasions, the cord injury is unilateral, affecting the lateral spinothalamic tract and pyramidal tract on one side only. The patient then presents with loss of pain and temperature-sensation on one side of the body, and limb weakness on the other—the Brown–Sequaard syndrome.

Examine muscle-power muscle-group by muscle-group if the patient is able to co-operate. In the unconscious patient, observe spontaneous movement or movement of the limbs in response to a painful stimulus. Examine the tendon reflexes in all four limbs, and attempt to elicit Babinski's and Hoffmann's reflexes. Following a complete cord injury the muscle tone below the level of the injury is usually flaccid, and the tendon reflexes absent initially.

Hypotension and bradycardia may be seen after complete cord injuries.

Spinal-cord injury

The great majority of spinal cord injuries occur at the time of
the accident; but an estimated 10 per cent of patients acquire

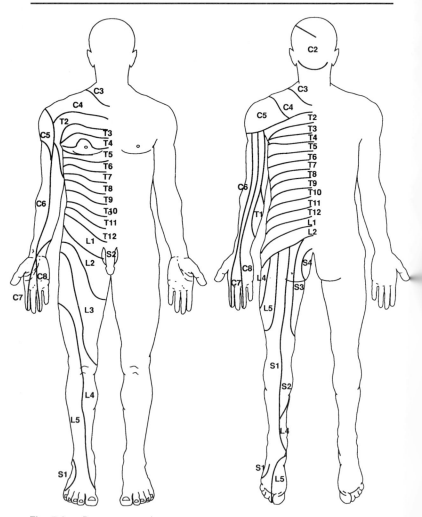

Fig. 7.2 • Dermatome charts.

a neurological deficit later as a result of further displacement of an unstable injury or cervical-disc herniation. If the spinal-cord injury is complete at the time of admission, with no movement and no sensation below the level of the injury, there is little chance of recovery. If the neurological deficit is partial, recovery is possible. In both cases it is essential that the spine should be stabilized in order to prevent further neurological damage and to enable recovery to take place if possible. In the case of the partial spinal-cord injury and in those patients with an unstable spinal injury neurological deterioration may take place, and must be recognized. Muscle-power and sensation must be tested at hourly intervals for the first 24 hours, and with reduced frequency thereafter. Progressive neurological deterioration may be due to swelling of the cord within a spinal canal narrowed by deformity, by vascular compromise, or by compression by disc material or haematoma.

Early management of the spinal injury

In the absence of a spinal-cord injury the stable spinal fracture should be treated with some form of orthosis. This may be a hard collar or a spinal brace, depending on the site and configuration of the fracture. Further, more detailed radiological examination may be required; and until this has been done the patient should remain horizontal. If the injury is thought to be unstable skull traction must be applied, and the patient should be placed on a suitable bed to allow turning without movement of the neck. If there is no cord injury the patient should be nursed on a Stryker turning frame. If there is a complete spinal-cord injury and an unstable spinal injury either a Stryker frame or one of a variety of tilting beds should be used.

Skull traction can be applied quickly and easily using the Gardiner–Wells skull tongs. The tongs are fixed to the skull by sharp pins which penetrate the outer table. The scalp is infiltrated with local anaesthetic 1 cm above the pinna on either side of the scalp. No incision or pre-drilling is required (Fig. 7.3).

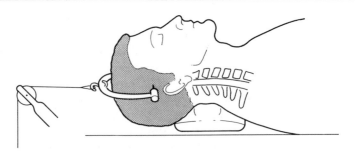

Fig. 7.3 • Application of Gardiner–Wells skull tongs.

When there is loss of alignment of the cervical spine due to fracture or dislocation early reduction is imperative, particularly when there has been progressive neurological deterioration. Skull traction should be applied in the resuscitation room under the supervision of an experienced Orthopaedic Surgeon or Neurosurgeon. The weight applied to the skull tongs depends on the level of the fracture. For a high cervical lesion 2.2–4.5 kg may be sufficient, whereas in the lower cervical spine 11.4–13.6 lb may be required. The X-rays should be repeated after traction has been applied, and after each increment until reduction has been achieved.

The injured spinal cord is sensitive to the same factors that cause deterioration in head-injured patients—hypoxia and hypotension. Early surgery for associated injuries must be carried out with great care, and every effort must be made to replace blood-loss and maintain adequate ventilation. The unstable spine poses particular problems for the anaesthetist during intubation and in subsequent positioning of the patient for surgery.

Various drugs, such as high-dose steroids, naloxone, and calcium antagonists, have been suggested as a possible means of reducing spinal-cord oedema after injury; but there is no convincing clinical evidence that these drugs bring about any neurological improvement.

Surgery has a very limited role in the early management of cervical-spine fractures. Decompressive surgery for spinal-cord injuries has not been shown to reduce neurological damage, and deterioration as a result of early surgery is well recognized. Surgery may be indicated for the stabilization of fractures or ligamentous injuries; but, in general, this is best delayed until the patient's general condition is stable and until it is clear whether the spinal-cord injury is complete. Urgent surgery should be reserved for those patients who show progressive deterioration due to spinal-cord compression by prolapsed intervertebral-disc material or haematoma. Early surgery is also indicated for unstable ligamentous injuries in the absence of a spinal-cord lesion, since these injuries tend to remain unstable unless some form of bony fusion is carried out. It may be very difficult to manage a restless head-injured patient who also has an unstable spinal injury and who is intent on getting out of bed. In these circumstances it may be necessary to consider an early spinal fusion in order to allow the patient to move around safely.

Further reading

Meyer, Paul R. (1989). *Surgery of spine trauma*. Churchill Livingstone, Inc., New York.

Shrago, G. G. (1973). Cervical spine injuries; association with head trauma: review of 50 patients. *American Journal of Radiology*, **118**, 670–3.

Chapter 8

Head injuries in children

Key points in head injuries in children

1 In the UK falling is estimated to cause 40–50 per cent of head injury in children.

2 The commonest cause of severe head injury in children is their running into the paths of oncoming vehicles.

3 In children subjected to physical abuse the commonest cause of death is head injury.

4 A head injury caused by shaking may present no outward sign of head trauma, but may be accompanied by a history of vomiting, fits, failure to thrive, lassitude, and irritability.

5 Where there is a history of trauma suspicion may be raised by an account inconsistent with the physical findings, the vagueness of the history, or an undue delay in seeking medical advice. Also by evidence of multiple injuries of different ages, or of neglect, and characteristic types of lesion: retinal haemorrhages, bruising in a fingertip pattern, and cigarette burns.

6 Radiologically, complex or multiple fractures, fractures involving more than one bone, and occipital fractures are suggestive of non-accidental injury, as are wide or 'growing' fractures and acute subdural and intracerebral haematomas and haemorrhagic contusion in the absence of skull fractures.

7 If a non-accidental cause is suspected the child must be admitted and an urgent consultation with a consultant paediatrician should be arranged.

8 In children under five conscious level should be assessed on the Glasgow Paediatric Coma Scale.

9 A 'growing fracture' (normally found in children under three) requires surgical repair in order to prevent the development of a skull defect that might render the underlying brain liable to injury.

10 *Contre-coup* cerebral contusions are rare in children, and should raise the possibility of non-accidental injury.

11 It is vital that information on the progress of a child with head injury is given to the parents consistently by a single senior person who is identified as being 'in charge'.

The epidemiology of head injury in children differs from that in adults, and the head injury in the child poses special problems of diagnosis, management, and rehabilitation.

The widespread belief that children, having youth on their side, are more able to tolerate and recover from head injuries than adults is erroneous. The developing brain is especially vulnerable to injury. On the other hand, children are less frequently injured as occupants of vehicles involved in road-traffic accidents, and thus tend to avoid the high-velocity head injuries so commonly seen in adults.

For the parents, the trauma of the child's injury is compounded by feelings of guilt, remorse, and anger. Since the parents may spend much of their time by the bedside of the injured child, other children in the family may be relatively neglected at a time when they most need reassurance.

Box 8.1. **Causes of head injury in children**

- Falls
- Road-traffic accidents
- Sports injuries
- Non-accidental injury

Causes of head injuries in children

The commonest cause of head injury in children is falling, estimated in various surveys in the United Kingdom as causing 40–50 per cent of children's head injuries. Falls occur in the domestic situation and at play. In infants, falling from chairs or changing tables is a frequent variety of accident. The incident is commonly not witnessed, and there is uncertainty whether the child had really fallen or not. Accidents at play are also often unwitnessed by adults, since they may occur out of doors, and the nature and severity of the blow is not known. Although domestic falls are common, and cause parents a good deal of anguish, they do not often result in severe head injuries. Resulting skull fractures from these mechanisms are usually closed linear fractures, and subsequent intracranial haematomas are uncommon.

Approximately 20 per cent of rear-seat occupants in the United Kingdom are children. Children are involved as passengers in road-traffic accidents, and their situation in the back seat does not diminish the possible severity of the trauma—indeed, there is evidence that back-seat passengers suffer more severe injuries than belted front-seat passengers. A study in the United States has shown an incidence of head injury of 70 per cent in children involved as rear-seat passengers in road-traffic accidents. It has been estimated that the use of rear-seat seat-belts could bring about a reduction of deaths in rear-seat passengers of 75 per cent. The compulsory use of seat-belts in the rear seats is expected to reduce severe injuries from this source. Children under the age of four years should be restrained in safety seats. Children over the age of four can be protected by standard seat-belts as long as a suitable booster cushion is used.

The commonest source of severe head injuries in children in their running out in front of vehicles as pedestrians. Children as young as four or five are regular victims, and lack of parental supervision plays an important part in the circumstances. These children suffer multiple injuries.

A British survey in 1991 found that 36 per cent of head injuries in children were due to road-traffic accidents.

Bicycle accidents are another common cause of head injury, and one which can also be reduced by safety measures such as the use of cycle helmets, the provision of cycle tracks, and the provision of cycling proficiency courses in schools. These head injuries are associated particularly with injuries of the cervical spine, upper limbs, and clavicles.

Non-accidental injury

It is important to be aware of the possibility that the injured child may be the victim of abuse. By its nature, the true incidence of this phenomenon is difficult to determine. One recent survey in England found that only 4 per cent of all head injuries in children were due to non-accidental injury.

In children subjected to physical abuse, the commonest cause of death is head injury. If the injury is caused by shaking there may be no outward sign of head trauma. In these circumstances the child may present with a history of vomiting, fits, failure to thrive, lassitude, and irritability. Where there is a history of trauma suspicion may be raised by an account inconsistent with the physical findings, the vagueness of the history, or an undue delay in seeking medical advice. On physical examination there may be evidence of multiple injuries of differing ages, the child may appear neglected, or the child's affect may be abnormal— withdrawn, frightened, or depressed. Retinal haemorrhages do not occur as a result of simple falls, and are well-recognized in association with non-accidental head injuries. Certain skin lesions are characteristic of physical abuse, and these include fingertip bruising (i.e. bruises inflicted by fingertips) and cigarette burns.

> **Be aware of the possibility of non-accidental injury.**

Certain radiological features increase the suspicion of non-accidental injury. Complex or multiple fractures, fractures involving more than one bone, and occipital fractures are highly suggestive. It has also been reported that wide or 'growing' fractures are characteristic of non-accidental head injury (see p. 136). Skull fractures in children, as in adults, may be complicated by extradural haemorrhage; but in the non-accidental injury subdural haematomas, intracerebral haematomas, and haemorrhagic contusion are common causes of neurological impairment and death. These lesions are often due to shaking, and may be found in the absence of a skull fracture. Their finding should raise the possibility of non-accidental injury.

If a non-accidental cause for the head injury is considered the child must be admitted to hospital, and urgent consultation with a Consultant Paediatrician should be arranged. A skeletal survey should be carried out in order to identify other injuries.

Box 8.2 **Clinical features of non-accidental injury**

- History inconsistent with physical findings
- Vague account of accident
- Delay in seeking medical attention
- Multiple injuries
- Child with abnormal affect
- Signs of neglect
- Characteristic skin lesions
- Retinal haemorrhages

Box 8.3 **Radiological features of non-accidental injury**

- Complex or multiple fractures
- Wide or growing fractures
- Occipital fractures
- Radiology inconsistent with history of injury
- Fractures of other bones & differing ages
- Subdural haematoma
- Cerebral contusion/intracerebral haematoma

Clinical assessment of the head-injured child

- Glasgow Paediatric Coma Scale

Exactly the same priorities apply to the resuscitation of the injured child as have been described for the adult. The neurological assessment, however, is complicated by difficulties of communication and co-operation in the younger child. In children over the age of 5 the adult Glasgow Coma Scale can be used to describe conscious level. In young children the recording of the verbal response must be modified, and in children too young to be able to obey a command the 'motor response' element must be modified accordingly. A modified Paediatric Coma Scale has been devised.

Box 8.4 Glasgow Paediatric Coma Scale

	>1 year	<1 year	
Eye-opening	4 spontaneously	spontaneously	
	3 to command	to shout	
	2 to pain	to pain	
	1 no response	no response	
Best motor response	5 obeys commands		
	4 localizes pain	localizes pain	
	3 flexion to pain	flexion to pain	
	2 extension to pain	extension to pain	
	1 no response	no response	

	>5 years	2–5 years	0–2 years
Best verbal response	5 orientated and converses	appropriate words and phrases	smiles and cries appropriately
	4 disorientated and converses	inappropriate words	cries
	3 inappropriate words	cries	inappropriate crying
	2 incomprehensible sounds	grunting	grunting
	1 no response	no response	no response

Normal aggregate score		
	< 6 months	12
	6–12 months	12
	1–2 years	13
	2–5 years	14
	>5 years	14

Radiological assessment

Linear skull fractures in children are no different from those seen in adults. In young children some fractures grow in width under the influence of raised intracranial pressure— in the presence of a subdural haematoma, for instance. The skull injury may involve unfused sutures, and present radiologically as a widened suture line. Depressed skull fractures in the young child with a soft pliable skull may present as **'pond' fractures**—saucer-shaped depressions rather like an indentation in a table-tennis ball. It may be difficult to gain the co-operation of a distressed or frightened child in order to obtain good-quality skull X-rays. It may be necessary to admit the child and defer further investigation until the child's confidence has been gained. The presence of a parent during the X-ray may be helpful. Because of the potential difficulties in obtaining a reliable history there should be a lower threshold for ordering skull X-rays in children.

The indications for CT scanning are the same as for adults; but it may be impossible to obtain a satisfactory scan in the restless or disturbed child. If the clinical indications are pressing, the child will require a general anaesthetic in order to carry out the scan.

Scalp injuries

The capacity for scalp lacerations to bleed heavily presents a potentially serious problem in small children, who can lose a significant proportion of their total blood volume from this source. Bleeding may also take place into the plane between the galea and the pericranium. The **subgaleal haematoma** forms a tense swelling extending from the forehead to the occiput. This may be extremely painful, and presents an alarming appearance. In the small child it may represent a significant loss of circulating blood volume. Unless aspiration of the haematoma is essential for pain-relief no specific treatment is required, and the haematoma will resolve spontaneously. Aspiration carries the risk of introducing infection—

potentially serious infection, with infarction of part of the scalp—and should be carried out with meticulous asepsis.

Skull fractures

Children's skulls are more pliable than those of adults, and may be deformed to a greater extent without fracturing. Linear fractures carry the same implications in children as they do in adults. The **pond fracture** referred to above may be disfiguring if it is outside the hair-line, but requires no treatment if it is within the hair-line and not associated with an overlying wound. The parents will need to be reassured that the palpable dent is harmless and will eventually disappear. If the fracture poses a cosmetic problem it is a simple matter to elevate the depressed portion of skull.

In a small proportion of young children with linear skull fractures there is a tendency for the fracture to grow. This phenomenon is rarely seen over the age of three years. As the fracture edges become more widely separated a skull defect is created. These are known as **growing fractures**. The reasons for this complication remain uncertain, but it is thought that it may be related to an underlying dural tear which allows herniation of arachnoid into the fracture. A growing fracture requires surgical repair in order to prevent the development of a skull defect which might render the underlying brain vulnerable to injury. The defect is explored and the underlying dural defect repaired. The fracture is repaired with a bone graft. In order to recognize this problem all children under the age of three years with substantial skull fractures should be reviewed as outpatients after about three months. Clinical examination of the fracture site is sufficient to exclude a skull defect, and only those with a clinical suspicion of a growing fracture need be X-rayed.

> **Children with large skull fractures should be reviewed after three months to exclude growing fracture.**

Intracranial haematomas in children

Extradural haematomas are seen in children, and present in the same clinical fashion as in adults. Whereas, in adults, 80 per cent of extradural haematomas are associated with a skull fracture seen on the skull X-ray, the incidence of associated skull fractures is lower in children—in the region of 60 per cent. This may be related to the greater elasticity of the child's skull and the greater adherence of the dura to the suture lines. Management of the child with a suspected extradural haematoma is no different from that in the adult; but there must be a greater readiness to admit the child with a head injury for observation, since one important indication of the possibility of extradural haematoma—the skull fracture—may be absent.

> **Children should be admitted for observation even in the absence of a skull fracture after significant head injuries.**

Acute subdural haematomas are not common in children, and should raise the possibility of non-accidental injury. **Chronic subdural haematomas** are sometimes seen, and are most common in children under the age of three years. In many instances, a history of trauma is not obtained, and the haematoma may be due to a relatively minor injury which has passed unnoticed. The history is usually one of irritability, vomiting, disturbed sleep and feeding patterns, and drowsiness and these children are less likely to present primarily to an Accident Department.

Contre-coup cerebral contusions are rarely seen in children, and, again, should raise the possibility of non-accidental injury.

Management of head-injured children

Head-injured children are more likely than adults to be admitted to non-specialist units for observation. In many instances, this will mean admission to a children's hospital separate from the adult hospital and the Neurosurgical department. An adult with the same injury might be considered worthy of admission to the Neurosurgical ward under the care of medical staff, and, more importantly, nursing staff, with specialist experience in the observation and management of the unconscious patient. The role of experienced neurosurgical nurses should not be underestimated, and there is a strong case for insisting that children with potentially serious head injuries should be observed in the early period of the illness in the Neurosurgical ward.

The parents are also patients.

The experience of having a child with a severe head injury is both terrifying and very distressing for the parents. Most parents will wish to remain in the hospital and at the bedside during the critical period. They will repeatedly seek reassurance from the medical and nursing staff, and from the physiotherapists and members of other disciplines, that their child is going to make a full recovery. At this stage, every hint of progress or deterioration is seized on; and it is vital that consistent information is given by one person, who is identified as being 'in charge'. This should be a senior member of staff. Apparent discrepancies in the information given increase the anxiety and, however unintentionally, give the impression that information is being concealed. In the case of the severe head injury, there are two stages to the process, and these should be explained to the parents. The first stage is the period when efforts are directed towards ensuring the child's survival; and at this stage it is usually impossible to give accurate information about the quality of recovery that might be expected. The second stage is the period of recovery and rehabilitation, during which the rate of recovery and the extent of possible recovery begin to become apparent. Care of the parents, the provision of simple factual information, and the availability of the doctor in charge of the child build a rapport that is essential in the long-term management of the head-injured child.

Further reading

Diagnosis and treatment of head injury in children. Youmans' Neurological surgery, Vol. 4.

Becker, D. P. and Gudeman, S. K. (eds) (1989). *Textbook of head injury*, Ch. 15: Paediatric head injuries—special considerations. Saunders, Philadelphia.

Hobbs, C. J. (1989). ABC of child abuse—head injuries. *British Medical Journal*, 298, 1169–70.

McLaurin, R. L. and Touban, R. (1990). Diagnosis and treatment of head injury in children. In *Neurological surgery* (ed. J. R. Youmans), pp. 2149–93. Saunders, Philadelphia.

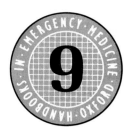

Chapter 9

Operative surgery

Key points in operative surgery

1 It is important to shave the scalp sufficiently to give a clear view of the surgical field, and to enable the wound to be extended if necessary. Surgical wounds should be planned so that they can be incorporated in more extensive scalp flaps should further surgery prove necessary after transfer to a specialist unit.

2 Bleeding from the scalp and extradural space can be heavy, so if anything more than a minor procedure is planned blood should be cross-matched in preparation.

3 The great majority of scalp lacerations can be closed under local anaesthesia with 1 per cent lignocaine and 1/200 000 adrenaline: but lengthy lacerations, scalping injuries and wounds involving skin loss should *not* be treated under local anaesthetic.

4 General anaesthetic technique should ensure that intracranial hypertension is not exacerbated during induction or in the course of surgery: the patient must be paralysed and ventilated, and *not* allowed to breathe spontaneously. Hypotension must be avoided so as to maintain adequate cerebral perfusion.

5 Once the patient is anaesthetized the endotracheal tube must be firmly anchored before the head is draped and the anaesthetist's access is obscured; the head should be supported on a head ring. A 30° head-up tilt of the operating table once the patient is anaesthetized helps to keep down intracranial pressure.

6 In ragged or contaminated scalp wounds care should be taken not to excise so much skin that the wound cannot be closed without tension.

7 In compound depressed skull fractures if the dura has been torn the laceration should be extended in order to inspect the brain and to remove foreign material, clot, and contaminated or devitalized tissue from it if necessary. Prophylactic antibiotics should be prescribed in all cases.

In the United Kingdom it is usually possible and desirable for head-injured patients requiring operative intervention to be transferred to a specialist unit. There are occasions when circumstances make this impossible, and the General Surgeon or Orthopaedic Surgeon may be required to operate in the District General Hospital. In many parts of the world the surgical management of head injuries is, of necessity, the responsibility of the General Surgeon.

In this chapter, those procedures that may be necessary in non-specialist units are described. Modifications to routine neurosurgical practice have been made, on the assumption that available equipment will be limited. Certain basic instruments are essential, and should be stored together as a craniotomy set.

Before embarking on cranial surgery certain principles should be borne in mind. It is important to shave the scalp sufficiently to give a clear view of the surgical field, and to enable the wound to be extended if necessary. Surgical wounds should be planned so that they can be incorporated in more extensive scalp flaps if further surgery may be necessary after transfer to a specialist unit. Bleeding from the scalp and from the extradural space can be heavy, and, if anything more than a minor procedure is planned, blood should be cross-matched in preparation.

Anaesthesia

• **Local anaesthesia** General anaesthesia

Local anaesthesia

The great majority of scalp lacerations can be closed under local anaesthesia using lignocaine 1 per cent and adrenaline 1/200 000. Lengthy lacerations, scalping injuries, and wounds involving skin-loss should not be treated under local anaesthetic, and these wounds should be cleaned and dressed and then left until the patient has been suitably resuscitated and prepared for a general anaesthetic.

General anaesthesia

It is beyond the scope of this book to discuss in detail the anaesthetic implications of head injury; but certain basic considerations should be remembered.

The anaesthetic technique should ensure that intracranial hypertension is not exacerbated during induction or in the course of the procedure. It is essential that the patient should be paralysed and ventilated, rather than being allowed to breathe spontaneously.

Hypotension must be avoided in order to maintain adequate cerebral perfusion.

During cranial surgery, the head may be moved, and there is a risk of displacing the endotracheal tube. Once the patient is anaesthetized the endotracheal tube must be firmly anchored before the head is draped and the anaesthetist's access is obscured.

The head should be supported on a head ring, so that it is stable and comfortably supported during the procedure.

When the patient's intracranial pressure is thought to be elevated it is advisable to tilt the operating table 30° head-up once the patient is anaesthetized. This helps to lower the intracranial pressure while preparations are being made to open the head.

Uncomplicated scalp laceration

Shave the scalp to give adequate exposure of the wound. Clean the surrounding skin with antiseptic solution and drape the area. Infiltrate the skin edges with local anaesthetic (but where there is any skin-loss a large volume of injected local anaesthetic can hinder approximation of the wound edges). Retract the wound edges and inspect the underlying skull for fractures.

In ragged or contaminated wounds the wound edge should be excised sparingly, taking care not to excise so much skin that the wound cannot be closed without tension.

Small wounds should be sutured in a single layer, using a non-absorbable suture material of gauge 3/0, such as nylon or silk or surgical staples. In large wounds it is preferable to carry out a two-layer closure, approximating the galea with absorbable sutures such as Vicryl, Dexon, or PDS and lightly approximating the skin edges with interrupted non-absorbable sutures.

Compound depressed skull fracture

Widely shave the scalp around the wound and position the head in the head ring.

Clean the skin with antiseptic solution, and drape the prepared area.

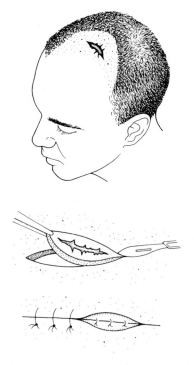

Fig. 9.1 • Suture of a scalp wound.

The wound is cautiously excised, taking care not to create a skin defect that cannot be closed without tension. Extend the wound in order to give a clear view of the fracture. A self-retaining retractor is inserted, and, in small wounds, this will usually ensure haemostasis. In larger wounds haemostatis is achieved by picking up the galea in artery forceps at 2–3 cm intervals and everting the skin edges. The artery forceps can be bunched together and retained by an elastic band.

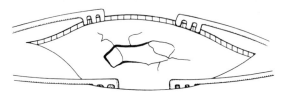

Fig. 9.2 • Exposure of a depressed fracture.

Having exposed the fracture incise the pericranium. A periosteal elevator is used to scrape the pericranium from the margins of the fracture.

The depressed bone fragments must now be elevated in order that the underlying dura can be inspected. It may be possible simply to lift out the fragments using bone rongeurs, but in many cases the depressed fragments are impacted. It is then necessary to fashion a burr-hole on the edge of the fracture so that an instrument can be inserted under the fracture.

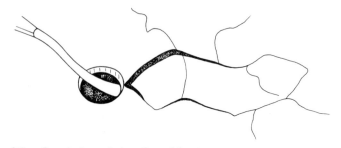

Fig. 9.3 • Burr-hole and elevation of fracture.

Remove the bone fragments and clean them by washing in a solution of **flucloxacillin** (500 mg in 500 ml normal saline), and set them aside. Foreign material is removed from the skull defect.

If the dura has been torn the laceration should be extended in order to inspect the brain. Remove foreign material from the cortical laceration. Clot and contaminated or devitalized brain are removed by gentle suction. Haemostasis can usually be secured by gentle packing with cotton-wool pledgets soaked in normal saline. Packing for 5–10 minutes is generally effective at controlling diffuse oozing. Alternatively, a layer of oxidized cellulose ('Surgicel') placed over the bleeding surface and covered with wet cotton wool is a very effective haemostatic manoeuvre.

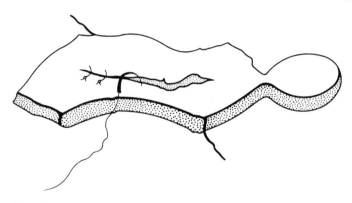

Fig. 9.4 • Dural laceration repair.

If the skull defect is small (2–3 cm diam.) the bone fragments may be discarded, unless this will produce a cosmetic blemish—which might be the case, for example, if the fracture were below the hair-line in the frontal area.

In larger defects the bone fragments are replaced. They may simply lie comfortably in place once the pericranium has been sutured; but larger fractures may have to be fixed with wire. Repair the wound in two layers using a 2/0 absorbable material to suture the galea and interrupted non-absorbable material for the skin.

Prophylactic antibiotics should be prescribed (see p. 000).

Procedures for extradural haematoma

- **Burr-hole and craniectomy   Craniotomy   When no extradural haematoma is found**

A burr-hole alone is of no value at all in the management of a solid extradural haematoma. Two procedures are here described for the treatment of this condition; but the ideal is to carry out a craniotomy.

The site of the haematoma is determined by the CT scan, or by the clinical signs if a scan is not available or clinical urgency precludes any further delay. The intracranial haematoma will cause a contralateral hemiparesis and dilatation of the ipsilateral pupil. The extradural haematoma is usually closely related to the site of the fracture, and the skull opening should be centred on the fracture site.

The proposed incision should be marked on the skin, and the scalp should be shaved. The head must be supported on a head ring. In order to prevent rotation of the neck the patient may have to be half rolled to one side and supported by sandbags. Rotation of the neck causes obstruction of cerebral venous return, and exacerbates intracranial hypertension.

Burr-hole and craniectomy

Infiltration of the scalp with lignocaine 1 per cent and adrenaline 1/200 000 reduces scalp bleeding.

A 7–8 cm vertical scalp incision is made within the hairline, and self-retaining retractors are inserted. The pericranium and temporal fascia are incised in the same line as the wound, and a periosteal elevator is used to separate the muscle from the skull. The self-retaining retractors are then replaced in this deeper plane, and the muscle is retracted. The fracture should now be evident.

A burr-hole is now fashioned, using first the perforato

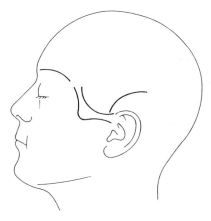

Fig. 9.5 • Scalp incision.

and then the burr attached to the brace and bit. The burr-hole is placed adjacent to the fracture, and care must be exercised lest the bit should slip through the fracture.

Having completed the burr-hole, the diagnosis will be confirmed by the sight of black haematoma extruding from the extradural space. Bright red blood is due to fresh bleeding caused by surgery, and does not represent haematoma! The bone defect must now be extended using a bone rongeur to enlarge the burr-hole until the margins of the haematoma are seen. Bleeding from the bone is controlled by bone-wax smeared into the skull margin.

The bulk of the haematoma can now be removed by suction or with forceps; but it is advisable to leave a thin layer of haematoma adherent to the dura, since this is providing haemostatis.

The dura should now be covered with a large piece of wet cotton wool, which, if left for 5–10 minutes, will stop most of the haemorrhage from the dural surface. The wool is then washed off with saline. A few bleeding-points may then be seen to persist, and these can be coagulated with monopolar diathermy or covered with oxidized cellulose.

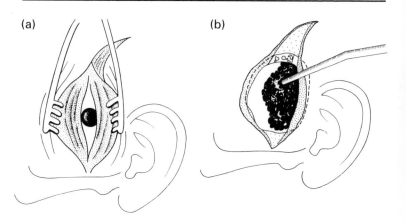

Fig. 9.6 • Burr-hole extended to make craniectomy.

Bleeding from under the bone edges can be controlled by suturing the dura to the pericranium at intervals.

Once absolute haemostasis has been achieved the pericranium and temporalis muscle are sutured. A suction drain is inserted in the subgaleal layer, and the wound is closed in two layers with 2/0 absorbable sutures to the galea and interrupted non-absorbable sutures to the skin.

The disadvantage of this procedure is that the skull defect will have to be repaired at a later date using artificial material. It does, however, have the attraction of simplicity.

Craniotomy

Depending on the site of the fracture, the scalp incision is planned in order to place the wound inside the hair-line and to ensure that the scalp flap retains an adequate blood-supply. Mark the proposed skin incision with an indelible pen.

Prepare and drape the scalp, and then infiltrate the course of the proposed scalp incision with lignocaine 1 per cent and adrenaline 1/200 000.

The surgeon and assistant compress the scalp against the skull by fingertip pressure while the incision is made in

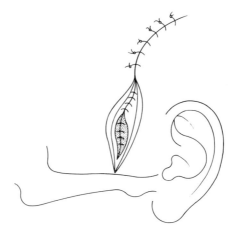

Fig. 9.7 • Closure of the wound.

stages. At each stage the galea is picked up with artery forceps and everted. The handles of the forceps are grouped together and retained by an elastic band.

Once the incision has been completed, the scalp flap is elevated by dissection in the plane between the galea and the pericranium or temporalis fascia. The skin flap is then wrapped in a wet swab and turned down on its base to expose the pericranium and temporalis fascia. Bleeding from the skin edges is arrested by diathermy coagulation.

The pericranium and temporalis muscle are incised using cutting diathermy, following the margin of the skin incision but leaving a broad pedicle at the inferior edge on which the bone flap will be reflected.

The pericranium is scraped back with the periosteal elevator, but should be left attached to the centre of the bone flap. Self-retaining retractors are used to spread the incision in the muscle on either side of the muscle pedicle.

At this stage the fracture should be evident. Burr-holes are fashioned at the four corners of the proposed bone flap using the Hudson brace and perforator, followed by the burr. Black clot may issue from the burr-holes, confirming the diagnosis.

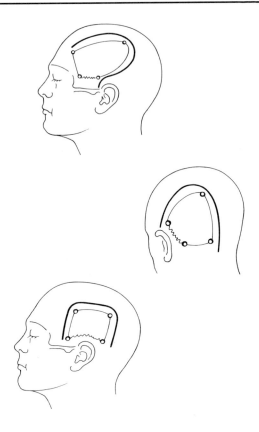

Fig. 9.8 • Examples of scalp incisions.

A blunt dissector (Adson's) is used to separate the dura gently from the skull at each burr-hole.

The saw-guide is passed in the plane between the skull and the dura from one burr-hole to the next, and the Gigli saw is threaded between the two holes. The saw handles are attached, and, by a steady to-and-fro action, the skull is sawed between the burr-holes. This is repeated at three sides of the proposed bone flap, while the inferior margin is left intact.

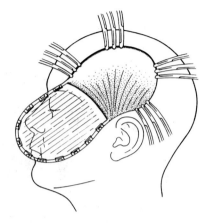

Fig. 9.9 • Fashioning the wound.

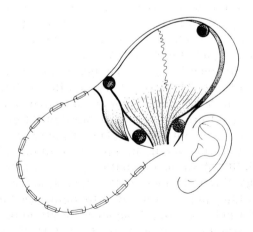

Fig. 9.10 • Incision in the pericranium.

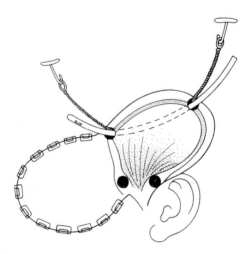

Fig. 9.11 • Fashioning the craniotomy.

A periosteal elevator is then inserted through the bone incision, and the bone flap is levered up until the remaining edge of the flap fractures, allowing the bone flap to be turned back. The bone edges may bleed, and this is controlled by pressing bone-wax into the cut edge of the bone.

The bone flap now remains attached to the skull by temporalis muscle and pericranium. It is wrapped in a wet swab, and reflected with the skin flap.

The extradural haematoma is now exposed as a mass of solid clot. The clot is removed by suction; but it is a good idea to leave a thin layer of haematoma on the dura in order to avoid provoking further dural bleeding. The dura should be covered with a large piece of wet cotton wool which is left undisturbed for 10 minutes. This allows diffuse oozing from the dural surface to settle, and leaves the main sources of bleeding to be dealt with. The cotton wool is then lifted off as the dura is irrigated with saline. Irrigation prevents the clot being avulsed from small bleeding-points.

Attention can now be turned to the main sources of haemorrhage. A common source is the middle meningeal

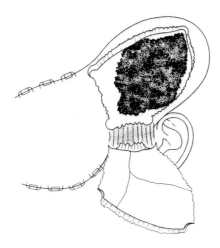

Fig. 9.12 • Elevation of a bone flap.

artery, where it is severed in the fracture. Bleeding from the artery is controlled by coagulation with monopolar diathermy. If the artery is injured in the skull base the bleeding is easily controlled by pressing bone-wax into the fracture or the foramen spinosum. This is much easier than using the old sterile matchstick referred to in some textbooks, and is usually more readily available! Other bleeding-points on the dura can be coagulated or covered with haemostatic gauze (oxidized cellulose or Surgicel).

Frequently, dural bleeding is found to be a diffuse ooze, and not to arise from a single meningeal vessel.

Bleeding from the extradural space under the edges of the craniotomy can be troublesome, and is controlled by sliding a piece of haemostatic gauze between the bone and the dura. If bleeding is heavy the dura can be hitched up to the skull by suturing it to the pericranium.

Once **all** bleeding has ceased the bone flap is replaced and held in position by suturing the pericranium with inter-rupted 2/0 absorbable sutures.

A suction drain is placed between the pericranium and the

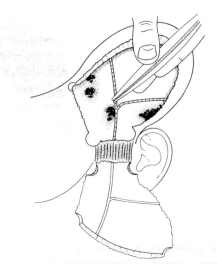

Fig. 9.13 • Coagulation of the middle meningeal artery.

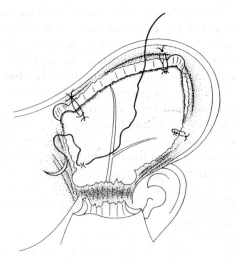

Fig. 9.14 • Hitching the dura.

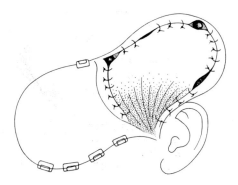

Fig. 9.15 • Suture of the pericranium.

skin flap, and the flap is replaced. The skin flap is sutured in two layers. Interrupted 2/0 sutures are used to approximate the edges of the galea, and the skin is closed with interrupted nylon or silk.

The head is bandaged. The drain is removed after 24 hours, and skin sutures are removed after 3 days.

When no extradural haematoma is found

Even when CT scanning facilities are available misinterpretation of the scan may lead to an erroneous diagnosis of extradural haematoma when the lesion is really subdural or intracerebral. In these circumstances no extradural haematoma is found, but the dura is tense and bulging. This creates considerable difficulty for the inexperienced surgeon, who must then decide whether to proceed to open the dura or whether to abandon the procedure and seek neurosurgical help. If the latter is not practical the dura should be incised and opened in a cruciate fashion. Obvious subdural haematoma may then be removed by a combination of suction and irrigation with normal saline. It should be remembered that the subdural haematoma is usually associated with a severe primary brain injury, and the underlying brain will be swollen. Unless the dura is closed rapidly the

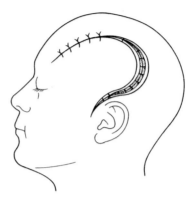

Fig. 9.16 • Closure of the scalp wound.

brain will tend to herniate through the craniotomy, and the wound will become progressively more difficult to close.

If surgery is thought to be necessary in the base hospital it is more likely that no CT scan is available to guide the procedure. If no extradural haematoma is found this may be due to incorrect location of the craniotomy, or to the fact that the haematoma is intradural. The craniotomy may be incorrectly sited if the haematoma is situated very anteriorly or posteriorly, or when the site of the skull fracture has been misinterpreted. In these circumstances the dura should be cautiously incised to identify a subdural haematoma, and if this is absent the wound should be closed and the patient should be transferred as soon as is practical to a specialist centre.

Further reading

Gudeman, S. K. (1989). Indications for operative treatment and operative technique in closed head injuries. In *Textbook of head injury* (D. P. Becker and S. K. Gudeman), pp. 182–191. Saunders, Philadelphia.

Keenan, Richard *et al.* (1989). Surgical anaesthesia in head injury. In *Textbook of head injury* (ed. Becker and S. K. Gudeman), pp. 182–191. Saunders, Philadelphia.

Symon, L., Thomas, D. G., and Clark, K. (eds) (1989). *Rob and Smith's operative surgery* (4th edn). *Neurosurgery*. Butterworth, London.

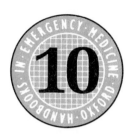

Chapter 10

Delayed complications

Key points in delayed complications of head injury

1 *Post-traumatic fits.* Anticonvulsants should be prescribed only if the patient has had a fit, and must then be continued indefinitely if the patient wishes to reduce the likelihood of recurrent fits. Phenytoin should be avoided in children because it causes gum hyperplasia, and sodium valproate in women of child-bearing age because of its teratogenicity. Phenobarbitone is more sedative than alternative drugs, and may cause hyperkinesia and behavioural disturbance in children.

2 *Meningitis.* The possibility of meningitis should be considered in patients who present with delayed symptoms weeks, months, or even years after a known head injury, especially a skull-base fracture. The characteristic physical signs are fever and neck stiffness, which may be accompanied by reduced conscious level and focal neurological signs such as hemiparesis or cranial-nerve palsies, and sometimes (usually later) papilloedema. Other common symptoms are progressive headache, neck pain, back pain, photophobia, and vomiting, and later drowsiness, confusion, and diplopia.

3 Except when there is any suspicion of an intracranial mass diagnosis should be confirmed, and the causative organism and its antibiotic sensitivity should be determined, by lumbar puncture. But when an intracranial mass may be present a CT scan should be ordered if available, or, if not, antibiotic therapy should be started *without* a lumbar puncture. (This course would apply for not fully recovered head-injury patients who might have intracranial haematomas or cerebral contusion and for those presenting with altered consciousness and/or papilloedema.) In these cases blood and any discharges should be taken for culture before therapy starts.

4 Immediate antibiotic therapy before the causative organism is determined should cover all likely pathogens: a combination of benzylpenicillin, cefotaxime, and metronidazole can be used. Therapy should continue for at least 2 weeks in the absence of a CSF fistula, or until any fistula has been repaired, with the lumbar puncture repeated if there is any doubt of eradication, and continuing therapy if a raised cell count persists.

5 Once the patient has made a full recovery from infection the possibility of a CSF fistula must be investigated, and if one is found it must be repaired, or there will be a risk of recurrence.

6 *Aerocele.* A large aerocele causes severe headache, usually of rapid onset, which may be accompanied by alteration of consciousness and focal deficits such as hemiparesis. Characteristically it occurs in a patient who has been recovering from head injury for some days or weeks, producing a delayed deterioration. Diagnosis is easily made by plain brow-up skull X-rays, which show the collection of air in the anterior fossa. They often resolve spontaneously; but this indicates there is a significant fistula which needs surgical repair to avert the possibility of meningitis. Antibiotic prophylaxis should be given.

7 *Hydrocephalus.* A rare complication, usually of severe head injuries. Clinical features include headache, intellectual impairment, urinary incontinence, and gait disturbance. Diagnosis is by CT scan, which may however also detect pre-existing symptomless hydrocephalus, not due to trauma.

8 *Chronic subdural haematoma.* Most common in the elderly and the alcoholic, and more likely in cases of cerebral atrophy. Patients present with headache, intellectual deterioration, focal neurological signs such as hemiparesis or dysphasia, and deteriorating consciousness.

9 *Subacute subdural haematoma.* More common in younger patients, with symptoms of persistent severe

headache and vomiting, nausea, and drowsiness, culminating in a final serious deterioration in conscious level.

10 *Post-concussional symptoms* (headache, dizziness, depression, lack of concentration, and lethargy) are diagnosed by excluding other, more serious, complications, since all these symptoms are found in other conditions. Impairment of short-term memory and concentration and depression can make return to work difficult, and the opinion of a Clinical Psychologist on the need for a period of convalescence can help to prevent the patient being regarded as a malingerer.

Delayed symptoms following head injury are common after both serious injuries and relatively minor injuries. Indeed, the delayed complication may constitute a much more serious problem than the initial injury.

Box 10.1 **Delayed complications of head injury**

- Post-traumatic epilepsy
- Meningitis
- Aerocele
- Hydrocephalus
- Post-concussional syndrome
- Chronic subdural haematoma

Post-traumatic epilepsy

- **Management of post-traumatic fits with anticonvulsant drugs**

Epilepsy may complicate both the relatively minor and the severe head injury. In the United States approximately 500 000 patients are admitted to hospital with head injuries each year, and 30 000 (16 per cent) have post-traumatic epileptic fits. An incidence of 5–7 per cent has been reported in European studies. This development should not be taken to indicate that some new and sinister intracranial event has occurred. It does not, for instance, herald an intracranial haematoma, and does not alone, therefore, indicate urgent admission to a Neurosurgical Unit. Post-traumatic epileptic fits are described as **early**, when they occur within the first week following the injury, and **late**, when they occur after the first week.

In the case of **early epilepsy**, 30 per cent occur within the first hour after injury, 30 per cent in the subsequent 24 hours, and the remainder in the following week. Of early fits 11 per cent involve an episode of status epilepticus, and in children under the age of five years the incidence is as much as 20 per cent. Early fits are more common after severe head injuries. A period of post-traumatic amnesia (PTA) of greater than 24 hours, depressed skull fractures, and intracranial haematomas are associated with an incidence of early epilepsy of 9–13 per cent.

Late epilepsy occurs in approximately 5 per cent of all head injuries. The likelihood of the patient developing late (continuing) epilepsy depends on the nature of the injury, and can be roughly predicted. The incidence of late epilepsy is dependent on age, the severity of the injury, the occurrence of early epilepsy, and complications such as intracranial haematoma and depressed skull fracture.

Box 10.2 **Factors associated with late epilepsy**

- Early epilepsy
- Severe head injury
- Age < 5 years
- Intracranial haematoma
- Depressed skull fracture

The occurrence of early epilepsy is associated with an incidence of late epilepsy of 25 per cent. If the head injury is complicated by extradural haematoma there is a 20 per cent risk of late epilepsy, and the risk rises to 50 per cent in the case of subdural and intracerebral haematoma. Depressed skull fracture is also associated with a high risk of epilepsy; but the risk is dependent on a number of other factors. Penetration of the dura, post-traumatic amnesia (PTA) of greater than 24 hours, and early epilepsy all increase the risk. The combination of PTA greater than 24 hours, dural tear, and early epilepsy carries a risk of late fits of more than 60 per cent. The severity of the head injury is defined by the duration of PTA. PTA of greater than 24 hours has a 25 per cent risk of late fits.

Some 50 per cent of late fits occur within one year of the injury; but a further 25 per cent present after 4 years.

There is usually little difficulty in recognizing a classical **grand mal seizure**, and this is the commonest form of **early** fit. On the other hand, **partial seizures** may occur—taking the form of focal motor fits or absence attacks. In the latter, the patient becomes unresponsive for brief periods of time, and this may be misinterpreted as a progressive deterioration in conscious level if the abrupt onset is not recognized. Late post-traumatic fits often have a focal element, involving involuntary movement, sensory disturbance, or dysphasia, depending on the site of the injury.

No specific investigation is required when the patient is known to have had a fit following a head injury. The diagnosis is based on the doctor's observation of the incident or the account of witnesses. An EEG is of little value.

Management of post-traumatic fits with anticonvulsant drugs

The management of fits in the acute phase of the head injury is described on pp. 64–6. Prophylactic anticonvulsant drugs have no influence on the development of late epilepsy. Anticonvulsants should be prescribed only if the patient has a fit, and must then be continued indefinitely if the patient wishes to reduce the likelihood of recurrent fits. The choice of drug is determined by the patient's age and sex. Phenytoin causes gum hyperplasia in children, and an alternative should be used. Sodium valproate should be avoided in women of child-bearing age, because of its teratogenic potential. The dose required in adults varies from one individual to another, and may have to be adjusted according to the success in controlling the fits and toxic side-effects. Doses in children are dependent on weight. Blood levels of phenytoin can be used to achieve therapeutic concentrations and to diagnose overdosage. They are unreliable for other drugs. Phenytoin, carbamazepine, and sodium valproate are the anticonvulsants of first choice. Phenobarbitone is an equally effective drug, but is more sedative than the others, and may cause hyperkinesia and behavioural disturbances in children.

Box 10.3 **Anticonvulsant drugs**

Phenytoin	200–300 mg/day
Carbamazepine	200 mg b.d., increasing to 800–1200 mg/day according to effect
Sodium valproate	600 mg/day in divided doses
Phenobarbitone	60 mg t.d.s.

Doses in children according to weight.

Meningitis

• Clinical features   Diagnosis   Treatment

Meningitis is a complication of the penetrating head injury and the skull-base injury. Penetrating injuries of the skull vault are usually clinically obvious, and if appropriately treated surgically are rarely complicated by infection. In the event of infection the commonest contaminating organism is *Staphylococcus aureus*.

Skull-base fractures are less readily diagnosed. CSF rhinorrhoea or otorrhoea may be clinically obvious or occult, and may appear to have ceased when, in fact, the fistula persists but the CSF is being swallowed. Since the fracture involves the paranasal air-sinuses or the mastoid air-cells a variety of organisms may be responsible for infection. By far the most common form of meningitis complicating head injury is the **pneumococcal meningitis** complicating fractures of the anterior fossa and the middle third of the face and fractures of the nasal bones. Prophylactic antibiotics are usually given for an arbitrary period after the injury or after the CSF leak has ceased. None the less, delayed meningitis may occur weeks, months, or years after such injuries, and the possibility of meningitis should be considered in patients who present with delayed symptoms after a known head injury.

Clinical features

The patient usually presents with a short history of progressive headache and *malaise*. Neck pain or back pain, photophobia, and vomiting are common symptoms. Drowsiness, confusion, and diplopia may follow. The characteristic physical signs are fever and neck stiffness, and these may be accompanied by reduced conscious level and focal neurological signs such as hemiparesis or cranial-nerve palsies. Papilloedema may be found, particularly in the later stages of the disease.

Meningitis frequently progresses rapidly, and there is a high mortality-rate, even when appropriate antibiotic therapy is started promptly. Early diagnosis is vital.

Diagnosis

Ideally, the diagnosis should be confirmed by lumbar puncture, and the nature and antibiotic sensitivity of the organism should be determined. A lumbar puncture should not be carried out if there is any suspicion of an intracranial mass, and, in these circumstances, a CT scan must be ordered first. This applies to patients with recent head injuries who have not fully recovered, and might, therefore, be harbouring an intracranial haematoma or cerebral contusion, and to patients presenting with altered consciousness and/or papilloedema. If scanning facilities are not available treatment must not be delayed, and antibiotic therapy must be started without a prior lumbar puncture. Before doing so blood should be taken for blood culture, and any nasal or aural discharge should be swabbed and sent for culture. A retrospective diagnosis may be possible if bacterial antigens can be detected by serology; but absence of bacterial antigens does not exclude the diagnosis of infection by a specific organism.

Treatment

As soon as specimens for bacteriological examination have been taken antibiotic therapy should be started. Until culture and sensitivity reports are available the treatment should cover all likely pathogens. When the patient is known to have had cerebrospinal fluid rhinorrhoea or an anterior cranial fossa fracture **benzyl penicillin** must be given intravenously in high doses (2.4 g 4-hourly in adults, and 180–300 mg/kg in divided doses in children). If there has been cerebrospinal fluid otorrhoea or a fracture of the petrous bone a variety of middle-ear commensal organisms may cause meningitis, including Gram-negative and anaerobic species. Treatment should commence with **cefotaxime** (2 g 8-hourly, 100–150 mg/kg in divided doses in children) and **metronidazole** (500 mg 8-hourly, 7.5 mg/kg 8-hourly in children). It is wise to give all three antibiotics in combination until the causative organism and its sensitivity has been established. Antibiotic therapy must continue until the infection has been eradicated, and until any cerebrospinal fluid fistula has been repaired. In the absence of a demonstrable CSF fistula antibiotic treatment should continue for at least 2 weeks; but if there is doubt about whether the infection has been eradicated the lumbar puncture should be repeated. If there is a persisting raised cell count in the CSF antibiotic treatment should continue.

Once the infection has been treated and the patient has made a full recovery the possibility of a cerebrospinal fluid fistula must be investigated. There is a risk of recurrent meningitis if the fistula is not repaired.

> **Treatment of post-traumatic meningitis includes repair of the skull-base fistula.**

Aerocele

Anterior-fossa skull-base fractures may be complicated not only by the escape of CSF, but also by air entering the anterior fossa. Since the brain may be adherent to the fracture site the air may form a 'balloon' in the frontal lobe, especially if air is blown in under force when the patient blows his nose. A large aerocele causes severe headache, usually of rapid onset. This may be accompanied by alteration of consciousness and focal deficits such as hemiparesis. Characteristically this occurs in a patient who is recovering from the head injury, and the deterioration comes days or weeks afterwards. In many instances a history linking the new symptoms to nose-blowing is not found, and the diagnosis is suggested by the nature of the original injury and the delayed deterioration.

The diagnosis is easily made by plain brow-up skull X-rays, which show the collection of air in the anterior fossa.

An aerocele will often resolve spontaneously; but this turn of events indicates that the patient has a significant fistula, which requires surgical repair to avert the possibility of meningitis. Antibiotic prophylaxis should be given.

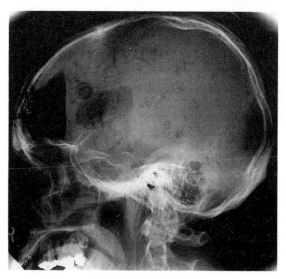

Fig. 10.1 • X-ray of an aerocele.

Hydrocephalus

Hydrocephalus is a rare complication of head injury. It occurs more commonly after severe head injuries, and may be a cause of delayed deterioration or arrested recovery. Blood in the cerebrospinal fluid may cause obstruction of CSF-flow in the basal cisterns, or failure of CSF reabsorption in the sagittal sinus. This results in communicating hydrocephalus. The patient may make an unexpectedly slow recovery, or cease to recover. Alternatively neurological deterioration may take place months or years after the head injury. The clinical features include headache, intellectual impairment, urinary incontinence, and gait disturbance. Papilloedema may occur, but is usually absent.

The diagnosis is made by CT scan. The finding of ventricular enlargement does not necessarily mean that the hydrocephalus is a result of trauma, however. Failure to recover as expected from a head injury may be due to pre-existing symptomless hydrocephalus, and treatment of the ventricular enlargement may not only be disappointing, but may also be complicated by acute subdural haematoma.

Chronic and subacute subdural haematoma

Chronic subdural haematoma is a condition which occurs most commonly in the elderly and in the alcoholic patient. In almost half these patients there is no previously recorded history of significant trauma. The pathophysiology of this condition appears to be related to venous haemorrhage from a bridging vein between the dura and the cortex. The possibility of this occurring is increased in those with cerebral atrophy and a greater interval between brain and dura. Instead of simply resolving, a membrane forms around the haematoma, and repeated haemorrhage from the highly vascular membrane leads to a gradual increase in the volume of the haematoma. The contents of the haematoma in the early stages are dark red, or black and tarry; but as time passes the fluid becomes dark brown, and then yellow, and more watery in consistency. Where there is a known injury, there is often a period of weeks or even months before the patient presents with headache, intellectual deterioration, focal neurological signs such as hemiparesis or dysphasia, and deteriorating consciousness. Particularly in the elderly or alcoholic patient, this diagnosis is worth considering in the event of delayed deterioration after a head injury—even a relatively trivial one.

In younger patients venous haemorrhage of this sort tends to present more acutely in the form of the **subacute subdural haematoma**. The patient who has had a relatively minor injury fails to recover from the initial headache, and continues to complain of nausea, vomiting, and drowsiness. Focal neurological signs may be absent in the early stages; but the patient's condition deteriorates over days or even weeks, culminating in a final serious deterioration in conscious level. The patient may have papilloedema. Drowsiness, focal neurological signs, persistent vomiting, and severe headache should make these patients readily distinguishable from those with post-concussional symptoms.

Post-concussional syndrome

- **Treatment**

Post-concussional symptoms are very common after head injury cause a good deal of anxiety among patients who have had minor concussional head injuries, and frequently lead to patients being reviewed in Accident and Emergency Departments or in the General Practitioner's surgery.

The most frequent complaints are of headache, 'dizziness', depression, lack of concentration, and lethargy. Each of these symptoms may be caused by other complications, and the diagnosis of 'post-concussional symptoms' is made by exclusion. Headache occurs in almost 70 per cent of patients who are admitted to hospital after minor head injuries (post-traumatic amnesia > 24 hours), and roughly 30 per cent of patients have headache that persists for more than 2 months. The headache is often related to exertion and fatigue, and is usually intermittent. Post-concussional headaches may be mild or severe. They are not accompanied by abnormal neurological signs. Dizziness is also a common complaint, and occurs in about 70 per cent of cases. True vertigo is rare. Some impairment of short-term memory occurs in a similar number of patients.

A careful history must be taken, with particular reference to symptoms such as rhinorrhoea, drowsiness and intellectual impairment, neck pain, photophobia, and vomiting. The patient should be re-examined and the X-rays should be reviewed. It is neither practical nor desirable to order CT scans for the large number of patients who present with relatively minor symptoms following concussional injuries. The likelihood of symptoms' being due to an intracranial haematoma is usually excluded by the time-scale. Extradural haematomas and acute subdural or intracerebral haematomas do not present after a delay of weeks, and almost invariably cause progressive neurological deterioration. Meningitis should also be readily recognizable from its characteristic symptoms and physical signs. In the elderly or alcoholic patient chronic subdural haematoma should be considered in the differential diagnosis, and there should be a greater readiness to order a CT scan in this group.

In the great majority of patients presenting with post-concussional symptoms, therefore, it is possible to make a clinical diagnosis and offer symptomatic treatment.

Treatment

The most important aspect of treatment is to explain the nature of the problem to the patient and to provide reassurance that the symptoms are not sinister, and will eventually resolve. Symptoms may persist for weeks or months. Depression may be responsive to antidepressant drugs.

Post-concussional symptoms may be associated with quite disabling intellectual impairment, although this may not be readily recognized on a cursory interview and examination. Impairment of short-term memory and concentration may make it very difficult for the patient to return to work; but the lack of obvious outward signs can lead to the patient being regarded as a malingerer. The opinion of a Clinical Psychologist can be invaluable in confirming that the patient is impaired, and should be allowed a period of convalescence.

Depression, anxiety, and lack of concentration may, on the

other hand, be due more to the cause of the injury—to an impending court appearance or a violent spouse. Post-concussional symptoms, by definition, complicate a concussional injury, and are not the consequence of an injury which has not resulted in even brief loss of consciousness.

Further reading

Friedman *et al.* (1945). Post traumatic vertigo and dizziness. *Journal of Neurosurgery*, **2**, 36–46.

Jennett, Bryan (1975). *Epilepsy after blunt head injury*. Heinemann Medical.

Rimel, R. W. *et al.* (1981). Disability caused by minor head injury. *Neurosurgery*, **9**, 221–8.

Soroker *et al.* (1989) Practice of prophylactic anticonvulsant therapy in head injury. *Brain Injury*, **3**(2), 137–40.

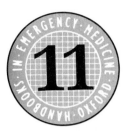

Chapter 11

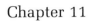

Transporting the head-injured patient

Key points in transporting the head-injured patient

1 Indications for urgent transfer to a neurosurgical centre are neurological deterioration; persisting unconsciousness (GCS 8 or less) *after* resuscitation; altered consciousness (GCS 9–11) and skull fracture; a focal neurological deficit; a compound depressed skull fracture; and a head-injured patient requiring ventilation. An early epileptic fit is not in itself a reason for transfer.

2 Chest X-ray, skull X-rays, cervical-spine X-rays, and arterial blood-gas analysis should have been performed before transfer, and blood-pressure and pulse-rate should be known, plus current status and any changes since the injury in conscious level (GCS) and neurological signs (e.g. pupil size, symmetry, and reaction to light).

3 In consultation with the neurosurgeon consider whether a diuretic (mannitol 20 per cent or frusemide) should be given before transfer, and whether endotracheal intubation and ventilation are indicated.

4 The patient *must* be stable in respiratory and cardiovascular terms before transfer.

5 In transport from the scene of the accident the airway should be cleared and if necessary protected with an oral airway; the patient should be transported semi-prone to avoid aspiration of vomit; and a high concentration of oxygen should be administered by face-mask. External blood-loss should be controlled by direct pressure, and the neck should be splinted in a rigid collar. Head-down tilting of the patient should be avoided.

6 Bleeding must be controlled and blood volume restored before transfer.

7 The unconscious patient must be monitored in transit by an experienced doctor, preferably an anaesthetist.

Pulse oximetry should be used in all transfers.
Intravenous anaesthesia and muscle-relaxants should be
administered by an infusion pump.

8 Any patient with a GCS of less than 5, or with
deteriorating conscious level, should be intubated and
ventilated before transfer.

9 A 500 ml bag of 20 per cent mannitol should be
available during transfer.

Secondary referral of head-injured patients

Following the primary hospital admission, resuscitation, and assessment, the head-injured patient may require referral to a Neurosurgical Centre or some other specialist unit in the acute phase. When dealing with the multiply injured patient it is essential to have a clear understanding of the indications for secondary referral, which may involve transporting the patient to a distant hospital, and is potentially hazardous.

Secondary referral is indicated if the patient has a severe head injury requiring intensive care under neurosurgical supervision, or a compound head injury requiring operative neurosurgical management. Transfer to a Neurosurgical Unit is required if neurological deterioration takes place because of intracranial pathology. It is important to remember that the commonest causes for deterioration are systemic factors—principally respiratory impairment and hypotension. Referral to a Neurosurgical Centre is also indicated if there are indications that the patient is at risk of developing an intracranial haematoma. Thus, the patient who has a skull fracture and remains unconscious (Glasgow Coma Score 11 or less) after resuscitation, and the patient who has a focal neurological deficit should have a CT scan. This often entails transferring the patient to a different hospital when scanning facilities are not available at the admitting hospital. Secondary referral may also be necessary for the management of other injuries when suitable facilities are not available at the admitting hospital. The most frequent example is that of the head-injured patient with a serious chest injury or facial injuries who requires assisted ventilation. Once the patient is paralysed and sedated no further clinical monitoring of the neurological condition is possible. An urgent CT scan is essential, and the intracranial pressure must be monitored in order to recognize an increasing intracranial mass in the form of a haematoma, cerebral contusion, or cerebral oedema.

An early epileptic fit is not in itself a reason for urgent referral, since this is not, in isolation, an indication that the patient has an intracranial haematoma.

Box 11.1 **Indications for urgent transfer to a neurosurgical centre**

- Neurological deterioration
- Persisting unconsciousness (GCS 8 or less) after resuscitation
- Altered consciousness (GCS 9–11) and skull fracture
- Focal neurological deficit
- Compound depressed skull fracture
- Head-injured patient requiring ventilation

Before the patient is transferred the neurosurgeon must be consulted, and the indications for transfer must be discussed. The neurosurgeon will require precise information about the patient's current condition and changes in conscious level and neurological signs that have taken place since the injury. Describe pupil size, symmetry, and reaction to light. Describe the conscious level at the time of admission and after resuscitation in the precise terms of the Glasgow Coma Scale. The blood-pressure and pulse-rate should be known. Describe any associated injuries. A chest X-ray, skull X-rays, cervical-spine X-rays, and arterial blood-gas analysis should have been performed. In consultation with the neurosurgeon, consider whether a diuretic agent (mannitol 20 per cent or frusemide) should be given prior to transfer, and whether endotracheal intubation and ventilation are indicated. The decision to transfer the patient and the arrangements for supervision in transit must be made by a senior member of staff.

Transporting the head-injured patient

- **Transport from the scene of the accident   Secondary transfer from the admitting hospital**

There are dangers lying in wait for the head-injured patient

> Box 11.2 **Information required by the receiving surgeon**
>
> - When did the injury take place?
> - What was the conscious level at the time of admission?
> - Has the conscious level changed since admission?
> - Are the pupils equal and reacting to light?
> - Are there focal neurological signs?
> - What are the blood-pressure and pulse-rate?
> - Has there been an episode of hypotension or hypoxia?
> - Is there any respiratory impairment?
> - Are the arterial blood gases normal?
> - Is there a compound head injury?
> - Is there a skull fracture?
> - Are there any other injuries?

both in the initial journey from the scene of the accident and in the journey from the admitting hospital to the specialist unit. There are approximately 6000 deaths as a result of road-traffic accidents in the United Kingdom each year. There is a high incidence of airway obstruction and serious blood-loss among those who die. Hypotension and respiratory insufficiency have a serious impact on the outcome of head injury, and measures that ensure efficient resuscitation at the scene of the accident and transfer to hospital increase the chances of survival. The introduction of Paramedics to ambulance services may contribute to improved survival in accident victims. In some parts of the British Isles, such as the Scottish islands or the North Sea oilfields, weather and distance combined with the need for air evacuation may cause delays of many hours.

Secondary transfer to a Neurosurgical Centre from the

admitting hospital may also involve several hours of travel by road ambulance or air. It is impossible to resuscitate the seriously injured patient in a speeding ambulance or a helicopter. It cannot be stressed too often that the resuscitation of the head-injured patient, however severe the head injury might appear, must be undertaken at the admitting hospital, and takes priority over all other considerations. The patient must be stable from the respiratory and cardiovascular point of view before being transferred.

A number of studies have shown a high incidence of extracranial insults occurring during secondary transfer. The commonest insults are hypoxia and hypotension, and these incidents are associated with significantly poorer outcomes and higher mortality. Similar observations have been made in intrahospital transfer (for example, for CT scan). Gentleman and Jennett (1981) reported that 45 per cent of unconscious patients transferred to a Neurosurgical Unit were inadequately resuscitated before or during transfer. Episodes of hypotension and hypoxia during transfer are more common in patients who have suffered similar insults prior to transfer. Complications during transfer have been shown to occur more commonly when the patient is escorted by a junior rather than an experienced doctor.

The head-injured patient must be resuscitated before transfer to a Neurosurgical Unit.

Transport from the scene of the accident

The principles involved in the transport of the head-injured patient from the scene of the accident are those that apply to all accident victims. The airway should be cleared, and then protected if necessary with an oral airway. The patient should be transported in the semi-prone position in order to avoid aspiration of vomit; and a high concentration of oxygen should be administered by face-mask. If the patient is making inadequate respiratory efforts after the airway has been cleared endotracheal intubation and assisted ventilation at the scene of the accident increase the chances of survival if suitably experienced personnel are present.

External blood-loss should be controlled by direct pressure, and the neck should be splinted in a rigid collar. Care must be taken not to throttle the patient with a tight cervical collar, since this raises the intracranial pressure. A record of the patient's conscious level at the scene may be an important indication of the severity of the primary injury.

The patient should not be tilted head-down as the stretcher is lifted into the ambulance or during the journey, and to avoid this the patient should be lifted head-first into the vehicle. Acceleration forces have been reported to cause reduction of cardiac output, and might, theoretically, have an adverse effect on intracranial pressure. A smooth journey at a steady speed is preferable to a very fast journey with periods of rapid acceleration and deceleration.

Helicopter transport is being used increasingly in some countries in place of road ambulances. There are a number of advantages in using a helicopter. Acceleration can be controlled more smoothly, and is only required at the beginning of the flight. A much less bumpy ride is possible. If the patient is transported feet-first, the effects of acceleration are counteracted by the nose-down tilt of the helicopter and the head-up tilt of the patient.

At all times be aware of the possibility of a cervical-spine injury, and ensure that the head and neck are controlled during movement of the patient.

Secondary transfer from the admitting hospital

Ensure that resuscitation has been completed. However severe the head injury may appear, the treatment of other injuries may take priority over the need to transfer the patient to a Neurosurgical Centre. In particular, any cause of respiratory impairment must be treated, bleeding arrested, and blood volume restored. This may mean, for instance, that a laparotomy is required to control intra-abdominal bleeding before the patient is transferred. It is quite clear from all the studies that have investigated inter-hospital transfer of head-injured patients that failure to stabilize ventilation and blood volume is associated with an un-favourable outcome.

The unconscious patient must be accompanied in transit by an experienced doctor, and not by the junior doctor who can most easily be spared. Ideally this should be an anaes-thetist. Monitoring in transit is just as important as it is before transfer. Manual recording of pulse and blood-pressure are difficult in a moving ambulance or in a vibrating military helicopter. Electronic monitoring equipment used in hospitals is often bulky and unsuitable for use in an ambulance, and some manufacturers supply compact units which provide ECG, blood-pressure monitoring, and oximetry in an easily portable form. Blood-pressure can be monitored by an automatic cuff such as the Dynamap; but intra-arterial monitoring is more accurate if a suitable monitor is available. ECG monitors vary in their reliability in an ambulance. Pulse oximetry should be used in all transfers. At the present time, suitably compact CO_2 monitors are not widely available.

Intravenous anaesthetic drugs and muscle-relaxants should be administered by infusion pump. This ensures a smoother and more predictable control of ventilation and intracranial pressure in transit.

The main hazards in transferring the head-injured patient arise from the possibilities of airway obstruction and im-paired respiration, continuing blood-loss, epileptic fits, and progressive intracranial haematoma in the course of the journey.

Venous access in transit
The patient should have a running intravenous infusion both for fluid replacement and for the administration of drugs. Since volume-replacement should have been com-pleted before transfer 0.9 per cent **saline** should be infused at a rate sufficient to keep the cannula patent. A 500 ml bag of 20 per cent **mannitol** should be available during transfer.

Epileptic fits in transit
If a fit occurs in the course of transfer the main concern is to maintain a clear airway. The fit itself does not call for any specific action unless it fails to terminate spontaneously in

2–3 minutes. In this event intravenous **diazepam** should be administered with great caution in small increments until the fit is arrested. There is a serious risk of causing respiratory depression if sedative drugs are given incautiously to head-injured patients.

Box 11.3 **Check-list before transfer**

Respiration	Is the PaO_2 > 13 KPa (100 mm Hg)?
	Is the $PaCO_2$ < 5 KPa (40 mm Hg)?
	Is the airway clear?
	Is the airway protected?
	Has the patient had a chest X-ray?
	Is intubation/ventilation indicated?
Circulation	Is systolic BP > 120 mm Hg?
	Is pulse-rate < 100?
	Is peripheral perfusion adequate?
	Is there a reliable i.v. line?
Head injury	Has the conscious level been recorded?
	Is the conscious level changing?
	Are there focal neurological signs?
	Is there a skull fracture?
	Is i.v. mannitol indicated?
Other injuries	Is there a cervical-spine fracture?
	Is there a chest injury?
	Is there an abdominal injury?
	Have major fractures been splinted?
Escort	Is there an experienced medical escort?
	Are essential drugs/equipment available?
	Are case-notes/X-rays available?

Care of the airway in transit

Respiratory inefficiency is potentially disastrous in the head-injured patient, and is very difficult to deal with in transit. If respiratory obstruction or deteriorating respiratory effort are anticipated the patient should be anaesthetized and ventilated before departure, and accompanied by an anaesthetist. The indications for ventilation depend on the distance that the patient is to be transferred, the experience of the doctor on the spot, the extent of associated injuries, and any history of prior respiratory impairment. Any patient with a Glasgow Coma Score of less than 5 should be intubated and ventilated before transfer. Any patient whose conscious level is deteriorating must be ventilated. This enables the intracranial pressure to be controlled until definitive treatment of an intracranial haematoma can be carried out. Although patients with severe facial or chest injuries may maintain adequate blood gases in the early stages there is a serious risk of deterioration in transit, and ventilation prior to transfer should be considered. There is a high incidence of hypoxic and hypotensive insults in transit among those patients who have had similar episodes prior to transfer, and consideration should be given to ventilation in this group.

It is important to make sure that the patient remains paralysed throughout the journey. This is achieved either by giving a continuous infusion of a muscle-relaxant by infusion pump or by intermittent intravenous boluses. Further neurological observation then becomes impossible, with the exception of the pupillary reflex, which is not affected by the paralysing agent. Ventilation can be continued manually by self-inflating bag, but is more conveniently maintained if a portable ventilator is available.

If a portable ventilator is to be used, the medical escort must be familiar with its operation, have a sufficient oxygen supply, and have equipment for hand ventilation in case of ventilator failure. Arterial blood gases should be measured before departure once the patient is established on the ventilator.

Transfer of the deteriorating patient

• Essential transfer equipment

The most important reason for transferring the head-injured patient to a specialist unit is neurological deterioration due to a suspected intracranial haematoma. Unless the surgeon at the admitting hospital has the experience and the confidence necessary to operate most patients are best served by being transferred to a Neurosurgical Unit. Since this may mean a journey of several hours' duration it is necessary to control the intracranial pressure temporarily until definitive treatment is possible.

Intubation and controlled ventilation not only prevent further deterioration due to hypoxia and hypercapnia, but, by lowering the $PaCO_2$, bring about a reduction in intracranial pressure. A rapid intravenous bolus of 20 per cent **mannitol** should be given while arrangements for transfer are being made. The dose is 0.5 g/kg body weight (i.e. approximately 200 ml for the average adult). This will 'buy' a period of grace of 2 hours at the most; so that no time should be lost in getting the patient moving. A urinary catheter should be passed, as a diuresis will occur as a result of administering the mannitol.

Box 11.4 **Transferring the deteriorating head injury**

- Ensure resuscitation completed
- Secure i.v. line
- Urinary catheter
- 20 per cent mannitol i.v. bolus of 0.5g/kg body weight
- Endotracheal intubation
- Ventilation
- Review pre-transfer check-list
- Immediate transfer

Box 11.5 **Essential transfer equipment**

- Oral airway
- Face-mask and self-inflating bag
- Oxygen cylinder and back-up cylinder
- Laryngoscope/endotracheal tube
- Portable suction machine
- Portable ventilator

- Selection of i.v. cannulae/giving set
- i.v. fluids—mannitol 20%
        —colloid solution (e.g. haemaccel)
        —0.9% saline
- ECG monitor
- Automatic BP monitor
- Pulse oximeter

- Drugs—muscle-relaxant (e.g. atracurium)
        —sedative agent (e.g. propofol)
        —diazepam
        —flumazenil
- Syringe pumps (battery-operated)

Further reading

Gentleman, D. and Jennett, B. (1981). Hazards of inter-hospital transfer of comatose head-injured patients. *Lancet*, **2**, 853–5.

Gentleman, D. (1990). Audit of transfer of unconscious head injured patients to a Neurosurgical Unit. *Lancet*, **335**, 330–4.

Gentleman, D. *et al.* (1981). Hazards of interhospital transfer of comatose head injured patients. *Lancet*, **ii**, 853–5.

Jeffries, N. J. and Bristow, A. (1991). Long-distance inter-hospital transfers [Helicopter transport]. *British Journal of Intensive Care*, **1**(5), 197–203.

Waddell, G. *et al.* (1975). Effects of ambulance transfer in critically ill patients. *British Medical Journal*, **1**, 386–9.

Wright, I. H. *et al.* (1988). Provision of facilities for secondary transport of severely ill patients in the United Kingdom. *British Medical Journal*, **296**, 543–5.

Index